Stories of San Diego

Stories of San Diego

A Collection About
People of Color and COVID

---

editor
Lindsay M. Hood

SD CWP

SAN DIEGO
CITY WORKS
PRESS

Copyright © 2024 San Diego City Works Press

All rights reserved. The authors retain the copyrights to their own works. No part of this book may be reproduced in any form without written permission from the publisher and/or the author.

ISBN 978-0-9837837-5-6
Library of Congress Control Number: 2024934576

San Diego City Works Press is a non-profit press, funded by local writers and friends of the arts, committed to the publication of fiction, poetry, creative nonfiction, and art by members of the San Diego City College community and the community at large. For more about San Diego City Works Press, please visit our website at www.cityworkspress.org.

San Diego City Works Press is extremely indebted to the American Federation of Teachers, Local 1931, without whose generous contribution and commitment to the arts this book would not be possible.

Cover image: Lindsay M. Hood
Cover design: Katareya Godehn Design
Production editor: Will Dalrymple | Layout & Editing | willdalrymple.com

Published in the United States by San Diego City Works Press, California
Printed in Canada

table of contents

Lindsay M. Hood
13   Introduction

community

Lindsay M. Hood
19   Barrio Logan—Follow the Vaccine

Nancy Shimamoto
27   Yonsei

J.W. August
43   COVID-19 Removes the Cloak Covering San Diego's Deep Ties to Racism

Paul Krueger
55   Alejandra Sotelo-Solis—The Mayor of National City Takes On COVID-19

Paul Krueger
61   Forging Trust—The Pandemic and San Diego's Black Community

Paul Krueger
65   Meet People Where They Are

Gabriella Rodriguez
71   COVID-19: The Most Powerful Border Wall Ever, A Binational Economic Killer

Will Huntsberry, Jesse Marx, and Bella Ross
75   The First Year of COVID: A College Degree Was an "Insurance Policy" Against Death

Brad Racino and Jill Castellano
83   Health Experts, Residents Worry South County Not Ready for Reopening As COVID-19 Worsens

Jill Castellano and Mary Plummer
97   Why Some COVID-19 Victims Are Dying at Home Without Medical Care

Jill Castellano
109   Remembering the Human Toll of COVID-19 in San Diego County

Jennifer Bowman
113   Even With Vaccines, San Diego's Vulnerable Communities Still Report High COVID-19 Rates

Roxana Popescu, Mary Plummer, and Jill Castellano
119   Coronavirus Deaths: San Diego Families Grapple With Mistakes, Slow Testing, and Poor Care

Jill Castellano and Mary Plummer
135   Uncounted: San Diego County's Pandemic Victims Far Surpass Official Totals

Will Huntsberry
147   The First Year of COVID: Farm and Construction Workers Among Those Most Likely to Die

MacKenzie Elmer
151   Volunteers Take Vaccine Appointments Door to Door in Barrio Logan

Maya Srikrishnan
155   The First Year of COVID: Filipinos Were Among Hardest Hit, But Hidden by Data

Maya Srikrishnan
165   Filipino Residents Have Been Hit Hard by COVID—But No One Knows Just How Hard

Maya Srikrishnan
173   Coronavirus Hit Latinos Harder Thanks to a Perfect Storm of Disparities

Kate Nucci
181   Black San Diegans Received a Quarter of All Coronavirus-Related Citations

Jesse Marx
185   On the Eve of Being Back on His Feet, He Was Gone

Maya Srikrishnan
191   Local Vaccine Rates Highlight Barriers Facing Black and Latino Communities

prison

Jill Castellano and Mary Plummer
201   County Jail Workers Prioritized for Vaccines While Inmates Have to Wait

Sofía Mejías-Pascoe
207   COVID-19 Cases at San Diego's ICE Detention Center Reach All-Time High

Jill Castellano and Mary Plummer
215   Donovan Deaths: 3 Prisoners Found Dead or Dying in Cells From COVID-19

Jill Castellano and Mary Plummer
223   Donovan Deaths: Families Kept in Dark While Inmates Die of COVID-19

Jill Castellano and Mary Plummer
233   *First COVID-19 Wrongful Death Claim Filed by Family of Donovan Inmate*

covid-19 hotels

Cody Dulaney
243   *San Diego County Won't Provide 24/7 Medical Services at COVID-19 Hotels, Despite SDSU Advice*

Cody Dulaney and Jill Castellano
251   *Problems Plague COVID-19 Hotel After County Pays Company Millions to Run It*

Cody Dulaney and Jill Castellano
261   *Scathing SDSU Report Says County Contractors Were Unqualified to Operate COVID-19 Hotels*

refugees

Roxana Popescu
273   *Pandemic Blew Open Digital Equity Chasm for San Diego's Refugees. What's Next?*

Roxana Popescu
283   *Pandemic Takes a Toll on San Diego County Refugees Sheltering in Place With Abusive Partners*

Roxana Popescu
291   *"It's Do or Die For Them." Life for San Diego's Refugees Was Tough. Then Came COVID-19.*

rent relief

Cody Dulaney
303   *Low-Income Tenants in San Diego County Can Get 100% of Past-Due Rent Erased*

Cody Dulaney
309   Hundreds Missed Out on Rent Relief When Landlords Didn't Take the Money

Cody Dulaney
315   Against Supervisors' Wishes, County Sent Rent Relief Money to Ineligible Cities

Lindsay M. Hood
Introduction

The color of one's skin is important and for some can be seen as a sort of currency. For some, the idea that some races can have an advantage seems ludicrous, but for many, just the smallest hint of melanin, a chemical the human body creates to protect itself from the sun, can have dire consequences.

How did we get to this point? Let's talk about racism and what it means. Racism is the power dynamic between the majority and minorities—the majority's use of power against minorities. We hear people talk about reverse racism, but without power and others who believe in the same ideals and stereotypes, reverse racism doesn't exist. At that point, it is just prejudice and bias. Race is a social construct. Every human has the same number of melanocytes. The more melanin these skin cells make, the darker you are; the less melanin, the lighter the skin color. Notice it is about skin cells not brain cells, but despite the science, entire cultures have been made to think otherwise.

According to Dr. Camilla Jones in her paper "Levels of Racism: A Theoretic Framework and a Gardener's Tale," racism is a system of structures, policies, practices, and norms that prioritizes opportunity and assigns value to a human body based on how much melanin your body produces. It is a system, not an individual character flaw nor a personal moral failing. There are three different types: institutionalized racism, internalized racism, and normalized or personally-mediated racism.

Institutionalized racism is defined as the differential access to goods, services, and opportunities by race. Institutionalized racism is normalized and can be legalized and may be manifested as inherited disadvantage. It has been codified into practice, customs, and law in both material conditions and in access to power. According to Jones, institutional racism includes differential access to quality education, sound housing, gainful employment, a clean environment, and appropriate medical facilities.

When it comes to health, only attacking institutionalized racism will create a profound change to affect structural conditions placed on minorities.

When COVID made its way to the North American continent, people were skeptical. How could bats sold in a market in an obscure province like Wuhan, China transfer the virus to humans in a "first-world" nation and pose any sort of threat?

But once the virus made its way onto the shores of North America and the rest of the world, institutionalized racism rumbled its way to the foreground. People living in first-world nations began making decisions for others across the world. Within first-world nations, it was between the haves and have nots. In the United States, if you were middle class or higher, with access to regular medical insurance, your life was a bit safer. The higher your class or status, the better off you were. But for people who fell below the middle class, healthcare was not always available, nor were the freedoms or access that America was built on.

Once COVID-19 shut down San Diego County, it was evident how imbalanced the system was. The people who essentially hold us up were falling down. They were deemed "essential workers," and their jobs had so much more meaning when we wanted Chinese food delivered to our house because we couldn't go out. All at once, everyone realized that the people who make our lives easier by handing us our mocha lattes through the drive-thru window were suffering. But did their lives become easier because of the realization? No, they merely got some memes on Facebook and claps at dusk. In real life, it was a different story.

For people of color, no matter the social class, COVID-19 was a reminder of where we stood in the moment. Everyday microaggressions became even more pointed and painful. Ohio State University's Monica Cox, Ph.D. points out that one of the ways institutionalized racism is visible is when policies and procedures put in place at companies only apply to certain people. Cox says when looking at those policies, look at who is given multiple chances, whose bad behavior is never addressed. In many workplaces, Cox says there aren't structures or systems in place where people of color feel safe and supported. Cox says no one wants an environment where people can't be themselves. All humans deserve to be in a place that accepts who they are and makes them feel safe. There is no reason people should die because they have no access to healthcare because their employers can't seem to find time to let them take time off to care for themselves or their families.

In this anthology, we look at people of color in San Diego and how they fared during the pandemic. We visit people and communities to see how they were affected.

community

Lindsay M. Hood
Barrio Logan—Follow the Vaccine

Tucked under the Coronado Bridge sits Barrio Logan. The neighborhood is surrounded by industry. To the west is San Diego Bay, the horizon dotted with Naval ships docked at Naval Base San Diego; shipbuilder NASSCO's enormous cranes jut into the sky ready to hoist steel beams over skeleton ships that will eventually flesh out into nuclear-class warships. To the North is downtown San Diego, a neighborhood littered with its own problems, like crime and homelessness. To the South is National City; Interstate 5 runs along the community's eastern border like a ribbon of concrete. Shiny cars pollute the air with exhaust and the steady hum from their engines.

The interstate splits into CA-75, which takes you into Coronado over the San Diego–Coronado Bridge. Over two miles of steel and concrete arch over the San Diego Bay. The onramp rolls right past the neon-lit sign which spells out Barrio Logan, each letter surrounded by a twinkle of lights to greet passersby. Every day, thousands of cars and trucks make their way back and forth across the girder bridge, which stands 200 feet at its highest point over the Bay to the Naval bases that call the island home.

Brightly colored murals adorn the columns of the bridge as it starts its course; the paintings depict stories and the struggles of Chicanos. The park in which these pieces sit is aptly called Chicano Park. According to Alberto Pulido, an ethnic studies professor at the University of San Diego and the co-director of the Chicano Park Museum and Cultural

Center, the park's existence is rooted in redlining, the practice that stopped people of color from moving into White neighborhoods.

Pulido says in the 1950s the neighborhood was multiethnic. According to a 1936 map from the Home Loan Corporation, neighborhoods from Barrio Logan and all the way east to Lemon Grove were marked as scarcely inhabited or undesirable. People of color who had moved to San Diego to work in the city's then thriving tuna industry were only allowed to live in these neighborhoods. They were not allowed to live in wealthier neighborhoods. Banks would not approve home loans in these areas for families of color. Some homeowners included language in the deed for their properties that the home could only be sold to Whites.

Pulido says it started to change in the late 1940s when Dr. Jack Kimbrough, San Diego's first Black dentist, started orchestrating sit-ins at hotels and restaurants demanding equal rights.

Pulido says Dr. Kimbrough was instrumental in ending segregation and bringing an end to redlining. However, the makeup of the communities was already set and remains in place today. People of color and the poor are still the predominant residents in these once redlined neighborhoods. Pulido says this made it easy for the state of California when they decided to build a highway in the early 1960s.

"You have a neighborhood that, prior to the building of the two highways, had 20,000 people living here, one of the largest Mexican neighborhoods in the state of California, only second to Los Angeles," Pulido said. "After the building of the two roads, we lose 75% of the community from 20,000 to 5,000."

Fast forward to March 2020 when the world started to shut down because of COVID-19. According to the San Diego Association of Governments, the 2020 population for Barrio Logan was 47,364, with 68 percent of residents identifying as Latino/Hispanic descent, 16 percent were White, 9 percent identifying as Black, and 4 percent identifying as Asian. The median income was $37,890.

In most communities, most tax dollars go to the wealthier neighborhoods. These residents have the time and resources to participate in local government and vocalize how they want their tax dollars spent. Wealthier citizens are also more likely to donate money to their favorite politicians.

Many people that live in Barrio Logan are low to middle income residents. The jobs they hold are essential to keep the economy going. Many residents work in the service industry or as day laborers. They are the people that make the world comfortable for the wealthy. The jobs are hard, require long hours, and result in very little pay, which means that they do not have time or wealth to get a politician's attention.

When COVID hit in March 2020, the community didn't have the same access to resources as wealthier neighborhoods. Enter the Chicano Park Steering Committee.

The Chicano Park Steering Committee was formed in 1970 by community members who wanted to preserve their neighborhood. After the state completed Interstate 5, dividing the community into two, the community worked to recreate and reclaim their neighborhood. The state, however, decided to build a California Highway Patrol station in the middle of the community, on the property that is now home to Chicano Park. The Chicano Park Steering Committee organized to stop the build. Ever since then, the group has worked hard to preserve its neighborhood and give its residents a voice. Lucas Cruz, a member of the Chicano Park Steering Committee, says the group has worked for 50-plus years making sure everything they do reflects what the community wants.

The community has come to rely on the committee as a resource. Cruz says, during the COVID pandemic, the committee stepped up to help provide resources to the neighborhood. When schools shut down, children who relied on free meals were able to continue to get food from the school district Monday through Friday. But the weekends were a different story. Cruz said, with many of their parents out of work, children faced food scarcity. The committee stepped in and distributed lunch to children on Saturdays at Chicano Park. The group distributed masks and hand sanitizer as well. When parks were able to reopen, the committee organized cleanups, and volunteers worked together to sanitize playgrounds, benches, and railings. Cruz says volunteers continue to clean bathrooms, keep up the cactus garden, and pick up trash without being asked.

Pulido says, for some residents, getting access to the vaccine was difficult. Barrio Logan residents lacked time and access. Many of the large public vaccination clinics organized by the San Diego County Department of Public Health were in wealthier neighborhoods. Pulido says that further cemented the fact that lower income communities do not always have access to healthcare. Doctor's offices are usually near hospitals in more affluent neighborhoods close to hospitals. Pulido said this is why Dr. Kimbrough was able to be so successful during San Diego's Civil Rights movement; his medical practice was in his own redlined neighborhood.

The problem of medical access for lower-income communities persists. COVID showed the inequities of healthcare not only in San Diego but also around the world. According to Pulido, the vaccine was not made readily available to the residents of Barrio Logan.

During the State of California's push for its citizens to get vaccinated, it created a website to help people find vaccination and testing sites. In wealthier communities with a communications infrastructure in place, this method worked. But in Barrio Logan, it became an obstacle.

According to Pulido, many people in the neighborhood do not have computers, are not computer literate, and do not have access to WiFi. Pulido calls it a WiFi desert. He says communications companies are not willing to come to their neighborhood because of barriers from the City of San Diego and the State of California, which owns the Coronado bridge. Many residents did not have the option to visit the State's website to get an appointment.

The County of San Diego's website was also difficult for some community members to navigate.

"It was like trying to get Comic-Con tickets. You get on there and, as soon as you try to get an appointment, it's gone," Cruz said.

The Chicano Park Steering Committee recognized the problem and set to work with other community groups to help residents get vaccinated.

"We didn't go out and ask whether groups would come and try to help us. We're taking the lead. We're working with another organization as partners to make sure that this comes to the community the right way," said Cruz.

The steering committee, however, did not have access to the vaccine and had to figure out how they could get access to it. Pulido said the lack of control in the distribution of the vaccine quickly became very evident. The County of San Diego's Department of Public Health was responsible for distributing the County's allotment from the State to qualified organizations, but the Chicano Park Steering Committee was not one of them. The committee had to look to another organization for help.

The marketing of COVID and potential to make money in a capitalist society did not go unheeded. Many groups saw COVID and its potential as a way to make money. For every vaccine given, it was money in their bank account. The steering committee shopped around and was able to find a group called the Champions for Health to supply and administer the vaccines to community members at their vaccination events.

The next question was where they could hold the vaccination events. The obvious place was Chicano Park, but Pulido had an idea to bring something familiar to the event to make residents comfortable. Pulido, who is the founder and chair of the University of San Diego's ethnic studies department, runs the department's community education program called Turning Wheel. The university provides the program with a large motorhome for students to work out of when they go out in the community. Equipped with a wireless hotspot open to the community, the motorhome is a familiar sight to residents in Barrio Logan who have visited the bus for access to WiFi. Pulido says they have dubbed it the "Barrio Bus." Using the familiar sight as homebase, the steering committee arranged three vaccination events aboard the Barrio Bus.

Each culture has its own way of communicating within its communities. When it comes to important information, Pulido says that, in Latino culture, getting verbal communication from a trusted source is key. While the plan was to have the community come to the Barrio Bus for their vaccine, getting the word out to the community that it was available would be the next hurdle. A long-time trusted community ally, the Brown Berets of Aslan stepped up to accept the challenge.

The Brown Berets have been working in the Chicano community for over 50 years, since the start of the Civil Rights movement. Pulido says the Berets are about protecting the community, stemming violence, and providing community support, similar to the Black Panther Party.

"When the pandemic first hit the community, I mean, Barrio Logan had really, really high rates of COVID," said Cheran Matewaay, a member of the San Diego Chapter of The Brown Beret National Organization. "Because a lot of our *gente* [people] there could not just stop going to work, could not just start working online or remotely, a lot of people were laid off."

The Berets started canvassing the neighborhood. They hung posters and started going door-to-door through the neighborhood informing residents about the vaccination clinics. A community hotline was created to help people find resources. Matewaay said they even made sure to talk to the unhoused living in the park so they could also have access to the vaccine.

Members of the Berets volunteered each day in front of the local Northgate Market's to sign up residents shopping at the store during the special COVID shopping hours for seniors. Matewaay says many then went to their regular jobs and then returned for a second shift in the evenings. The Berets worked to sign up people who might have otherwise been forgotten.

In the first week, the Berets were able to sign up 400 people for its first vaccination event. By the time of the event, its vaccine provider only had 300 doses to offer. As Pulido pointed out, it was a lack of control and something else they had to try to prepare for. But they created a waiting list to make sure everyone had an opportunity.

The group was able to put on three separate vaccination events and vaccinated about 1,000 people just by canvassing the neighborhood.

"Day laborers, essential workers, people who had to ask for time off from work," Pulido said. "I had to sign papers to prove that they actually had to come here because their employers wouldn't let them come."

Many residents in Barrio Logan did not have the luxury of choosing where they were able to work. Matewaay said people were not able to just start remote work. "It's a really big privilege to be able to just get your laptop and work from home."

A lot of people in the area were laid off, so unemployment became a huge issue for the neighborhood. People were sick and losing their jobs on top of it.

"It was pretty devastating, I would say, for a lot of people. A lot of us knew a lot of people who had passed away and a lot of people that were sick," Matewaay said.

The Brown Berets put up signs across the community offering help through a special hotline staffed by volunteers. The group also created a resource list so people would not have to repeatedly look up the same information.

"We put signs around the community saying if you needed help during the pandemic, give us a call," Matewaay said. "We would try to connect them with whatever they needed."

"How do I get free diapers? Where is the closest food bank I can go to? How do I sign up for unemployment?" Those were some of the most common questions the hotline fielded, according to Matewaay.

Despite their best efforts, loss and grief still rippled across the community, but the work brought a community together, and the future is bright.

"I think we need to look forward and celebrate all this important work, celebrate life, celebrate what we're doing because, you know, there's a lot of good. There's a lot of good that has come from this," Pulido said.

Nancy Shimamoto
Yonsei

My name is Nancy Shimamoto, and I live in San Diego, California. I'm a bit of an oddity because I am a fourth-generation Japanese American, or Yonsei. All of my grandparents were born in Hawaii, which makes them second generation, or Nisei. My parents were Sansei, third generation, also born in Hawaii.

In 2020, anti-Asian hatred and violence were front and center. The community held rallies, protests, forums, panels, and press conferences to attest our united desire to stop the hatred.

I don't know what caused this latest outcropping of severe violence against Asians. Perhaps it was partially due to our former president, who used racial slurs, unsubstantiated accusations, and supremacist rhetoric to engage his base. Fueling the fire of distrust was COVID, sheer anger, and suspicion of new mask mandates and gathering guidelines.

People who are intolerant of those who look "different" seem to embrace these opportunities to hate. And I think they've been given the right to hate, not just Asians, but a lot of minorities in the U.S. Black and Brown communities, Native American communities—we're all suffering more hatred than before.

I feel a lot of the anger and resentment is targeted to newer immigrants, and I hope these newcomers are forming or joining organizations to understand what is happening in America today. Together, we can all speak up, as a group in solidarity, because it is really important right now. We cannot let this hatred go unchallenged.

It's not like we've been given gifts once we got to America; we all worked very, very hard for what we achieved. The myth of the "model minority" has been concocted to drive a wedge between Asians and other minorities, forcing us further apart from each other, fomenting continued hatred for each group. This has got to stop, and efforts by the aforementioned groups are attempts to repair damage.

2020—The Year of Lockdown

Like all of the U.S., I spent 2020 in lockdown, for the most part. No visits with family, no in-person church worship, concerts, travel, or public events—Pride Parade canceled. My husband and I got through it, celebrating Thanksgiving with one relative, safe within our pod. We managed to have a semi-merry Christmas, though nothing about it was familiar to us.

We, along with many friends and acquaintances, were tired and fed up with the lockdown. We understood the reason for it; however, we were impatient and ready to move on. After a non-celebratory New Year's Eve passed, news of vaccine availability started to spread. Finally something to look forward to, if one could only score an appointment at UCSD's parking lot venue downtown, and get there on time, after fighting vaccine gridlock.

2021—The Year of Living Dangerously

We were fully vaccinated in early 2021, thanks to our new home in a continuing care retirement community. We moved here in March 2021 after coming for our vaccines and seeing the beautiful facility. Residents are 99 percent vaccinated, employees, 97 percent vaccinated. Our own little herd immunity! We thought we were safe and protected in our bubble, but we found ourselves frightened to travel, as COVID has reached four fully vaccinated people in our community. Anti-Asian rhetoric could be heard on the news and in the streets where it is whispered, sometimes shouted.

Even before 2021, I had heard of anti-Asian violence swirling throughout California and other states. It was devastating to see old people being pushed down to the ground, kicked, and beaten to death. Trump's "China Virus" rhetoric had turned the nation against all Asians, and we were feeling the hatred in our communities. Then, Atlanta happened. Six Asians slayed by one White man, along with a Hispanic and White person. Eight people were killed in a matter of minutes. The killer "had a bad day" according to a reporter. The killer pleaded guilty to four murders; charges on the other four are still pending. None is categorized as a hate crime.

After Atlanta, news of Asian American Pacific Islander (AAPI) hate crimes became widespread (increasing by 70% over 2020 statistics). Some in my church family felt fear, increased anxiety, and didn't leave their homes after this tragic event. We held a healing circle for the Asian Americans in our congregation. Non-Asians were allowed but politely asked not to speak. I took a class on hate crime intervention—what to do if I see another person of color being harassed, or worse. Still, I felt sheltered from the anger, as I had not experienced any direct animosity towards me.

Then it happened. At a gathering in our common courtyard, a woman sitting next to me used the term "China Virus," and I immediately asked her to "please, don't use that phrase. It is very hurtful to some people who are Asian Americans, whether they are Chinese or not." "I lived in China for 6 years, and everyone knows they spread it." "It's the COVID virus, not the China Virus," I insisted. Her response? "Every virus is COVID." Rather than continue arguing truth from fiction, I stood up, walked away, and sat at another table. I've spent hours thinking about how someone could blatantly ignore my request to stop using a hateful term, while looking me straight in the eye. I felt defeated, resentful, hated. I have not recovered from that encounter, mild as it was, compared to some of my friends' experiences.

Has COVID affected my life? Of course it has. Although I'm fortunate to not have close relatives die of this virus, I know plenty of people who have lost loved ones. I know chaplains who have been with the dying, as their families could not enter the room. We've all given up our freedom, missed family reunions, weddings, births, deaths. Just when we thought we were safe to move about again, the Delta variant grabbed center stage and now ravishes the unvaccinated and even some of us who are double-vaccinated. It's not fair, and it causes me great anger and distress to think we're repeating the nightmare of last year with rising cases, hospitalizations, and deaths. Because this virus and its prevention was politicized back in 2019, we are woefully short of the vaccination rate needed to create herd immunity.

Evidence shows the COVID-19 virus originated in Wuhan, China, although it is still unclear if it escaped from a lab or was transmitted by wild animals. The unfortunate use of hateful rhetoric to describe it, such as the China Virus, or the Kung Flu, has raised suspicion of Asian Americans (with all of us lumped into one category, regardless of myriad Asian ethnicities). I believe these uninformed ideas contributed to newfound prejudice against the Asian American community, which has been targeted with suspicion, racial bias, hate crimes, and sometimes murder. It is infuriating.

My Story

People my age are mostly Sansei, and kids, maybe 30 or 40, are the Yonsei. But being fourth-generation, I grew up with grandparents who all spoke English, so I speak no Japanese other than what I learned in college.

My grandparents and my great grandparents lived in Hawaii for quite a while, and then they came over to the U.S. mainland, I believe in the 1920s, somewhere around there. They went to the Los Angeles area and established some farmland that they leased. And eventually my dad's side of the family moved to Imperial Valley where they farmed in Brawley.

My grandfather, since he was an American citizen born in Hawaii, was able to buy land in Imperial County, California. So he bought acres of land to start farming there right next to the Westmoreland Cattle Ranch.

My mom's family went to Santa Maria, California, north of Los Angeles, farming strawberries up there for quite a while.

The term "Jap" makes my blood run cold. I've never gotten over being called that name in elementary school or reading the words in my mother's diary she kept during incarceration by the U.S. government. I don't imagine White folks understand the amount of discrimination Asian Americans have endured since we first immigrated to the U.S. If they knew, how could they continue the hatred and bias that has long plagued us? Attack us with microaggressions, even when we politely ask them to stop? I've inherited the pain and insult that my parents endured while incarcerated as American citizens. It is part of my DNA, just like the color of my skin, the shape of my eyes. How do I deal with it? I talk about my story to those who will listen and work to make positive change for all immigrants to the U.S., I hope.

"Camp"

It is finally becoming a well-known fact that 120,000 Japanese Americans were "interned" in relocation camps located away from the West Coast, due to fear they were communicating and colluding with Japanese warships. They were thought to pose a threat to the U.S., even though a majority of them were American citizens. So, Executive Order 9066 was issued on February 19, 1942, ordering people of Japanese ancestry to evacuate from the West Coast to these incarceration camps. My family learned of EO 9066 on April 1, 1942 and made plans for their evacuation. My maternal grandparents from Santa Maria drove down to Imperial because they wanted to be close to their daughter, now married to my dad and living on the Shimamoto family farm.

Somehow, my paternal grandparents were able to rent their farmland to local growers during their absence. They were greatly aided by their neighbors, the Westmoreland family, who agreed to keep an eye on the property, farm equipment, and belongings. The Westmorelands were family friends; I have photos of their kids and our uncles and aunts and kids growing up together. They were lifesavers and remain family friends to this day.

My mom kept a diary from the beginning of evacuation, that she allowed her three daughters to read. Unfortunately, it was lost over the years, so we no longer have that to refer to. But I have clear memories of some of her accounts, especially from evacuation day. My mother wrote in her diary, saying they had a month to gather their things and prepare for evacuation. They were allowed to take one suitcase per person on the bus and they were told to report to the main highway at 6 AM on a hot day in May 1942. My family went directly to Poston, Arizona, (unlike San Diego families who went to Santa Anita Racetrack, where they were held from April to August 1942, waiting for their barracks to be built). They stopped in Indio where they were fed a box lunch and then went on to Poston, arriving around 5:00 PM.

When they first got there, my mom said they were given a mattress cover and told to stuff it with straw for their beds. That was after being on the bus for the entire day. She said that was just the last straw (literally!) and she broke down and cried. And it was just heartbreaking.

Poston is in the middle of the Arizona desert on Native American land. It was very, very hot. There was little privacy, especially in the latrines, which brought further shame on the women. Curtains took the place of walls in the barracks, so they just had to learn to deal with everybody else right on top of them, which was very unpleasant for them. She said the food was terrible when they first got there, and if they got fresh fruit, they would save it for the children. Eventually, incarcerees took over the kitchens and produced food that was deemed edible to their families.

Windstorms were really pervasive in the desert, blowing sand and debris everywhere. Every time they had a big windstorm, it would blow off the roofs of the barracks, and the men would go out and collect the wood to make furniture. So there are a lot of pieces of furniture that were made by people who knew how to do woodworking. Many are preserved at the Japanese American Historical Society of San Diego (JAHSSD).

Life in camp was hard for the adults; but they were so innovative and resourceful, forming groups to manage vegetable farming, building kitchens so they could cook their own food rather than getting government rations, education, recreation (they even built a swimming pool for the kids), entertainment, newspaper production; the list goes on and on.

While in Poston, Arizona, she gave birth to my oldest sister, Dale. There was a huge labor shortage due to the war, so some JA (Japanese American) internees were allowed to leave camp and go into Utah or Colorado to farm. My family went off to harvest crops in Colorado and then returned to camp once the harvest season was over.

While farming in Colorado, my mother took Dale to a park to play. A woman told her "Japs aren't welcome here! Get out!" I can't imagine the hurt my mom felt that day, and every day ,during and after incarceration.

The day-to-day effort to live in the barracks was exhausting. In the book *American Concentration Camps*, my mom spoke of their friend Roy Westmoreland, who visited them, bringing with him lifesavers such as washing machines, a baby buggy, and a baby bassinet.

"The washing machines were truly lifesavers. I had been washing, rinsing, and wringing the heavy sheets and diapers by hand, and in the heat it was very, very hard," my mother said during the interview. When Mr. Westmoreland learned that mom had given birth to my sister Dale, and was hand-washing diapers, he literally brought the washing machine out to Poston camp and gave it to my mom, so they could use it for the laundry.

Mr. Charles Westmoreland passed away in 2017 at the age of 89. My sister Gwen went to the funeral in El Centro where she thanked his family for the kindness they showed our family and other Japanese in the valley during the war.

Freedom From Barbed Wire (The Other Lockdown)

In 1947, when the war ended, Japanese American families were allowed to return to their homes. Unlike my family, who had angels protecting their land, many JAs returned to nothing: houses taken over by White families, farms decimated of crops and equipment, stores and businesses looted and ruined. You see, in the 1900s, Asians were not allowed to own land unless they were American citizens, and most could not become American citizens.

Around the turn of the 19th century, anti-immigration sentiment was rampant, especially immigration from Asian and non-European countries. The U.S. Immigration Act of 1924 prevented Japanese immigration, and the Alien Land Law prohibited land ownership by aliens of Asian ancestry. Non-U.S. citizens were prohibited from purchasing and leasing land, and Asians were not allowed to become American citizens.

My grandfather actually owned his land because he was an American citizen, born in Hawaii, so my family was able to return to the farm and resettle there. But there were other JAs who were not allowed to own land prior to the war, so they leased their land and had no say over it. So when they went back, it was uncertain that they could start farming again. My grandfather helped get leases for farmers in the area when they returned. I'm really proud of him for that gesture of kindness.

My family resettled on the farm, while my Aunty Margaret went to Chicago to meet up with her husband, James Matsumoto, who served in the army's famous 442nd K company, which rescued the "Lost Battalion" in France. K Company started with 200 men and returned with 8. For his bravery, my uncle received a Bronze Star and a Purple JHeart for combat in Italy.

My dad's brother, Edgar, was in Minneapolis, serving in the MIS interpretive services for the U.S. Army. His wife traveled with Aunty Margaret to join Edgar. Eventually, they all returned to the family farm and joined my grandfather's Shimamoto and Sons farm, keeping it going until 1995.

My mom and dad returned to the family farm and worked hard to build homes for themselves and my uncles. My sister Gwen and I were born in El Centro and grew up with many cousins within a mile radius. Dale and Gwen attended a one-room schoolhouse located on the Shimamoto farm. By the time I was ready for kindergarten, our family had moved to San Diego due to my father's health. He suffered a heat stroke while building my uncle's home and had to get out of the intense heat of the Imperial Valley.

My dad started a little plant nursery, Bob's Garden Supply on Imperial Avenue in San Diego, which supported our family for about 10 years. He then went to work for the Retail Clerk's Union at Safeway as a produce manager, while my mom continued running the nursery. She was interested in horticulture and studied to become the very first certified nursery WOMAN in California! She then went on to work for Presidio Nursery, owned by another JA family, the Asakawas.

In elementary school, I was bullied and taunted for being Japanese ,and my mother, the brave soul that she was, went down and talked to this kid's parents, and after she did, I never heard another word out of this kid about my being Japanese.

So I really thank her for her bravery in standing up for us. My folks made a lot of sacrifices—a lot—to allow us the least discrimination possible. I believe her ultimate sacrifice was giving up her Buddhist religion. Both my mom and dad grew up in Buddhist families and practiced Buddhism as kids and as adults. But when they returned from incarceration, and my sisters were old enough to attend school, she made the decision to convert us to Christianity. Her reasoning? "We were already different enough."

She wanted to spare us from the prejudice of not being Christian in a majority Christian country. She felt Christianity was a bedrock of America and refused to make us appear "un-American" by practicing Buddhism. As with most things, there are silver linings, and my parents both became very strong Christians, raised us as Christians, and to this day I am still very active in the United Church of Christ. While I am grateful for this gift, I loathe the reasoning behind it: to spare us from additional prejudice due to our religion.

Looking back, it was a horrible sacrifice for them to make: converting from Buddhism to Christianity not because they thought Christianity was a better religion, but to save us from appearing "un-American."

My church, Pioneer Ocean View United Church of Christ, is an Open and Affirming, multicultural church in Clairemont. Ocean View United Church of Christ, which started out in 1920 as a Japanese church, was where my family converted to Christianity. Services were held in both Japanese and English, and almost everyone was Japanese American.

Fifteen years ago, we merged with Pioneer Church, an Anglo church with an aging population. So we came together and bonded as one church, one of only a few successful mergers of a multicultural church. To address this anti-Asian hatred, our pastor, the Reverend Mary Sue Brookshire, has been working very hard to give us a platform on which to speak, on which to heal, and to inform our sibling congregation about what we've been through.

Even as co-congregants, all worshiping God, we don't understand each other. So we are trying to use this opportunity to let everyone understand our backgrounds, where we've come from, how we've gotten to where we are, and how we are *us*. It's a long painful story for many people, and some have yet to share their stories.

My sisters and I all graduated from college and had successful careers in business and teaching. I worked as a product marketing manager for Hughes Aircraft Company, and my middle sister was a teacher. My oldest sister was an accountant. In my career, I was able to travel the world, where I was often the only woman in a room of industry leaders. I was received as a professional and respected manager in European and Asian countries, never subjected to sexist or racial bias. Unfortunately, I can't say that about my American counterparts and bosses here in the U.S. My favorite customers were in Japan, where I always received a genuine welcome and developed professional relationships with my counterparts, some of which continue today.

Back on the farm, my grandfather and uncles struggled to keep Shimamoto and Sons profitable. Their main crop was asparagus, but they also grew cantaloupe and some citrus. Asparagus was their cash crop, even though it required extra care due to the intense heat of the valley. They developed a very elaborate cooling system for the asparagus: a big hydrocooler, which took the just-harvested asparagus down to low temperatures, preserving it for shipment to specialty markets, like Gelsons in LA. Eventually, the crop was devastated by this thing called the asparagus aphid, and they just didn't have the money to do the big spraying that would wipe it out. So they eventually started selling off their land, and by 1995 they had basically disbanded, having leased or sold the land to others to farm.

I don't think things changed a whole lot for the family once they all returned to the valley. They didn't express bitterness or anger. I think part of my father's silence came from anger, but he never expressed it. My mom was asked how she felt about evacuation and, if I may read again from the book, she said, "We don't dwell on the past. We sometimes feel that some good must have come from this experience and we do not feel bitter. Sometimes bitterness is another word for self-pity." I think it represents what a lot of the people did post-war. They picked up and tried to move on with their lives as best they could.

Of course, those memories never disappeared; they left a permanent scar, but JA parents tried to lessen the negative impact on their kids. I think they wanted to save us from the shame and hurt that they had endured through the experience.

I do remember my mom speaking about the intolerance of other Americans when they went to Colorado, and my sister wasn't allowed to play with their kids. And they were very cruel, very outspoken about not wanting Japanese people around them. But as for the government, I don't recall either one of them ever expressing anger at the U.S. government.

My dad was reluctant to talk about incarceration. I don't remember having a conversation with him about it. My mother was a little bit more vocal, and she was actually interviewed for the book referenced above, *America's Concentration Camps*. She gave some information about what it was like to live in the camps, how she felt after returning to the farm, and how the experience had affected her. My grandparents seldom responded to questions, but I recall my grandmother saying that people had scavenged their home, even stealing photos of her parents hidden behind the wallpaper. To this day, we don't know if it was the FBI, or farm workers who lived in their house when they were incarcerated, who ransacked their home.

It is unfortunate that we haven't heard more stories directly from those who experienced incarceration under a U.S. order. In the years following the war, 60-70 years ago, people who were incarcerated were very ashamed, even though they knew that they had done nothing wrong.

This shame of being stripped of everything and being put into a prison camp paralyzed them from protesting or even sharing the experience afterward. I'm not sure any of them came to terms with it at that time.

It wasn't until their Sansei children started asking questions and forcing their parents to talk about it that the truth was finally shared and heard. These brave lawyers and civic leaders demanded answers from both their parents and the government. It is what started the movement towards reconciliation and reparation between the people who had been incarcerated and the U.S. government. Eventually, after long legal and political battles, on August 10, 1988, the U.S. Congress passed House Resolution 442, or "An Act to Implement Recommendations of the Commission on Wartime Relocation and Internment of Civilians," awarded restitution payments of $20,000 to Japanese American survivors of World War II civilian internment camps. It was assigned Public Law No. 100—383."

Preserving Our History

Some internment camps have been preserved and sit on National Park land. Poston Memorial, located on the Colorado River Indian Reservation is commemorated with a monument. Manzanar is designated a National Historic Site and includes a beautiful interpretive center, along with preserved buildings and sites. Tule Lake National Monument recognizes the camp where JAs, deemed "potential enemies of America," were taken, segregated from their families.

The San Diego Japanese American Historical Society (JAHSSD) is instrumental in preserving our history in San Diego. They house a huge archive of pre- and post-war artifacts and documents in their City Heights location. The Japanese American Citizen League (JACL) is a national organization, whose ongoing mission is to secure and maintain the civil rights of Japanese Americans and all others who are victimized by injustice and bigotry. San Diego has three JA-affiliated religious groups, many of whose members are active in human rights and interfaith issues. They, along with other non-profit organizations, work hard to address current and past JA and Asian issues here in San Diego. I am proud that the JA community stood arm-in-arm with our Muslim siblings as they faced discrimination, hatred, and violence after 9/11. I work with JAHSSD to tell my story, as a 4th generation JA, educating the public about JA incarceration during WWII.

Thank God we've been given an opportunity to express ourselves if we so choose. I'm extremely thankful that I can express what it's like to be an Asian American who has lived in this country since my birth. I'm in my early 70s. I've never thought about living anywhere other than the United States; my family has been here for four generations, so we belong here, and we call it home.

I don't think anybody should challenge us on that. I believe that we have been too quiet for too long. We have been raised to keep our heads down, work hard, don't say anything negative, don't rock the boat. We've been very good at that.

It's ironic that somebody would tell me, an American who's been here for four generations, to go back to where I came from. I've probably been here a lot longer than them, and yet I don't have the "right look." So I think it is now terribly disturbing and very unfair to the immigrants who have come seeking asylum or a better life, paying their way the whole time for it.

This is our home—whether we've been here one year or for hundreds of years—and I think it's very important that the different organizations in the Asian American community continue to have rallies, continue to meet, and continue to offer opportunities for us to speak out and be heard. Now is the time to stand up together, even though Asian America is made up of many, many different ethnicities. We stand now as one group, and we have to make sure that we let others know what we stand for and that we are not about ready to pick up and go someplace else.

So yes, like I said before, there's always a silver lining, if we search hard enough. My silver lining is an opportunity for me to tell my story and have it be heard. I am extremely thankful for the opportunity that America has given me and my family, even though my family was literally torn apart simply because they were Japanese Americans. We continue to work hard, continue to be educated, and continue to give back to the communities in which we live.

J.W. August

COVID-19 Removes the Cloak Covering San Diego's Deep Ties to Racism

Racism's effect on our community and on our lives was never made more visible than during the early months of the pandemic, especially during the protests against the death of George Floyd, which combined to create a volatile San Diego region.

The rejection of institutions and the demeaning of different racial and political groups bubbled up in a perfect storm that swept through the country and was fanned by the pandemic and political scapegoating.

What happened in our community can be better understood if you understand San Diego's history of racial tension. Like other metropolitan areas of the country, racism was always part of the fabric of our region as it grew in size and influence.

The Klu Klux Klan emerged in the 1920s in San Diego, as a rebirth of that "secret" organization that targeted Blacks in the south. The San Diego Klan was also an anti-immigration group that targeted new arrivals from foreign countries, along with Blacks and Jews. San Diego Klan No. 64, as it was called, met in a large hall in North Park, near Idaho Street and University Avenue.

"These histories of hate are deeply embedded into San Diego," Danny Avitia, a political activist, student, and a sociology major at San Diego State University told me. Avitia believes that the unrest in the spring and summer of 2020 was the "direct result of race relations and class struggle in America."

The reemergence of the Klan and with White supremacy, which continues to this day, is the basis for extremists' actions, according to San Diego journalist and hate group expert Brooke Binkowski. Neo-Nazi, Atomwaffen Division, Western Hammerskins, and San Diegans for Secure Borders are some of the active groups according to the Southern Poverty Law Center, which tracks hate groups in California and across the country.

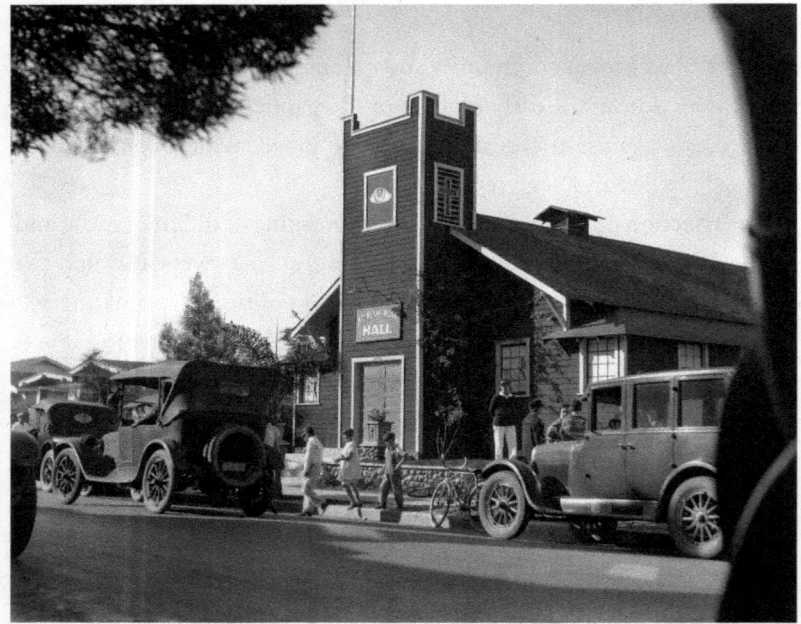

Photo courtesy of the San Diego History Center

The events of that spring, Binkowski said, prove once again the groups might change names or leaders, but they always adhere to the same goals and use the same tools of misinformation and fear.

"They spread stories about immigrants carrying diseases," Binkowski said. "They spread stories about immigrants doing crimes, especially Black immigrants."

In 1934 hate crimes were rarely reported, including when a number of Mexicans were found dead in lemon groves along El Cajon Boulevard, some disfigured by torture. The crime was explained in detail during congressional hearings. The transcripts from the 1934 Subcommittee of the Special Committee on Un-American Activities, 73rd Congress, 2nd session paint a vivid picture of life in San Diego.

The report revealed local newspapers refused to investigate cases of Klan hatred for fear it would create a bad image for San Diego.

In the late 1970s and the early 1980s, Ku Klux Klan leader Tom Metzger, a TV repairman from Fallbrook, joined with a neo-Nazi and former grand wizard of the Knights of the Ku Klux Klan, David Duke, in a series of publicity stunts to "protect the border." Metzger created an offshoot called the White Aryan Resistance in 1983 that evolved over the decades into the White Aryan Movement with the same White supremacist dogma. These groups, in turn, provided the impetus for the current crop of White supremacist patriot groups in Southern California, and here in San Diego.

The popularity of the internet and social media platforms have heated the rhetoric and hatred, allowing even small fringe groups to grow in prominence by attracting like-minded followers," Binkowski said. "There's now this poisonous rhetoric that is causing people to go over the edge; they're being convinced that the government is lying to them. With social media, you're able to kind of communicate with one video, to a whole movement. And social media really made this happen."

Avitia agreed, saying that before the street protests began, Black and Brown Americans knew they were hit hardest by the pandemic. The lopsided numbers showing the differences between races angered many, he says. This was just another form of discrimination as has happened for years, and the police killings only added fuel to the fire of anger and distrust, Avitia said.

This discrimination "is kind of normal life for us," Avitia said. "For Mexican Americans, for Black Americans, we deal with this all the time."

The most visible evidence that triggered serious rioting in La Mesa was when a White police officer arrested a Black man at a transit center, in La Mesa, California on May 27th, 2020, two days after the murder of George Floyd in Minneapolis.

Matthew Dages, an officer with the City of La Mesa's police department, arrested Amaurie Johnson. The arrest was captured on video by both Johnson's friends and a police body-worn camera. Johnson's arrest drew a strong and immediate reaction when video was posted on social media showing Dages grabbing and pushing Johnson onto a concrete bench.

Officer Dages would later be charged with one felony count of lying on a police report about the incident, though a jury later found Dages not guilty of that alleged perjury.

Within days, protestors took to the streets of La Mesa to protest the way Johnson was treated. On May 30, 2020, a protest began at La Mesa police headquarters, and by the end several businesses were looted and some torched and burned to the ground. Estimates of the number of people involved varied, but it's generally agreed that more than 1,000 people were involved.

"When the federal government did not act with a coherent plan for COVID, it created a vacuum, and into this stepped the racists," said Rasahanna Lee, who helped organize protests through this tumultuous period and used both Twitter and Instagram to recruit and tell others what she was seeing. Lee also marched with Black Lives Matter on the streets of San Diego and said she believes "the federal government relinquished its responsibility" when it didn't act.

Lee believes that led to a series of sometimes violent protests of various sizes across the community. It struck her how powerful social media was in encouraging others with an interest in social justice to be part of the effort.

Social media platforms also fed the "other side" of the issue, Binkowski said, as those right-wing groups used their agendas for chaos and as a means to rile up other protestors. It gave those involved "permission to act on their most craven impulses," she said.

Lee and Binkowski say they witnessed repeated efforts by the Proud Boys, a White supremacist group, to use the unrest as a way to push their agenda and recruit members. For example, Lee says she saw "a lot of courting of anti-vaxxers by the Proud Boys" during a protest in Pacific Beach, even though she said she thought "the anti-vaxxers appeared not motivated by hate but more by a common mistrust of government."

"These were well-dressed White people, who were publicly claiming that the COVID virus was grown in a lab and that the government was using it in an effort to control your mind," she said.

Binkowski described the protestors as "very White, they're very privileged, they can afford, you know, medical care for their children. COVID drove their racist attitudes."

Reporter Dave Summers of NBC 7 was covering the protests and noted some of the same things. He too saw White supremacists at every Black Lives Matter protest he covered. Summers says the other protests by anti-maskers seemed to have participants who were very passionate about their belief the country was going in the wrong direction. "It seems to be more of this in affluent communities," he said. Summers added, "I got a lot of flack from people." He recalled one instance where he met a young woman "who was very caustic about the whole thing and called us [the media] sheep because we wore masks and were not willing to engage in any escalation of the protest."

Avitia, who is gay, said White supremacy is embedded into gay and LGBT culture. The different groups within the gay community are as splintered as the heterosexual world is over race and pandemic issues.

"You should be in your own gay community," he said by way of example. "You shouldn't be with the lesbian community; the lesbians should stay with lesbians."

There are lesbians who have Nazi tattoos as well as gay men "who believe Whites should stay with Whites only, Mexicans stay with their Mexican gay folks," Avitia, said.

Focusing on the efforts of the Black Lives Movement during the protests and rioting was San Diegan Henry Wallace, a Black Panther with a keen interest in the group's efforts. He is an entertainer, a singer of "soul music" classics, something he began as a young man in the Bay Area. He remembers clearly how as a teenager he and his brother were in downtown Richmond, California looking for outfits for his fledgling band when a riot broke out. He saw "people were running, and the police were up on the roof shooting down at them." He said, "We ran and hid in a funeral home, and after all the shooting stopped we went home, and my mother was beside herself." Wallace's mother was upset. She said, "Here my kids are in the middle of a riot, something I have never seen." The family moved to San Diego, a "safe haven" for his mother and the family. Wallace's sister enrolled at what would become San Diego State University, joined the Black Student Union, and became politically active. That activism eventually led her and her boyfriend, Kenny Dimon, to reach out to the national chapter of the Black Panther Party, which approved their request to organize a local chapter of the national party in San Diego. "I joined because of the trauma that I went through up in Richmond and what I saw had happened at Watts," Wallace recalls. "I knew that I had to get in because it was open season on Black folks."

Wallace credits the Panthers with educating him about being an American citizen and teaching him how to handle run-ins with "White racist police" in San Diego. "I was taught a certain vocabulary when encountering the police."

Now, older and, he says, wiser, Wallace hopes the lessons he learned as a Black Panther can translate to the Black Lives Matter movement. In his time, "we were rushing to right wrongs, not taking the time to evaluate every step," which hurt the group's efforts, he observes.

Wallace thinks the Black Lives Matter movement has similar challenges.

"It's fast moving, so there are going to be missteps," he said. The protests are a valid tool to express anger over injustice, Wallace said, but, he warned, "other people came in and disrupted our movement by being violent. If you have an activist organization you have to monitor, and analyze your internal operations; if not, you will have problems."

He counsels the protestors to "get savvy, get politically active" because "power does not give up power. You have to work on it and move it slowly but surely."

Media coverage during the spring of 2020—and later—was 24 hours per day, seven days a week at the national and local level as widely diverse agendas all fed the public's anxiety. San Diego was facing the same quandary as Americans everywhere—who can you trust, they wondered? The protests, fights, and uglier incidents like the burning down of businesses all reflected the widespread fear, anger, and confusion of the time. San Diego had more traditional media lining up against right leaning television, websites, and radio. KUSI, One America News, and talk show programs on AM radio appeared to support the Trump agenda, describing certain protestors as "un-American." The local NBC, CBS, ABC, NPR, FOX affiliates in San Diego, I was told by numerous sources within different newsrooms, wrestled with how best to provide coverage that honestly reflected the dynamics in play.

Along the fringes, groups normally hidden from the mainstream rose in prominence, representing the extremes of both sides. Into the breach came the reporters who were tasked with telling the story, often at great risk to their own safety—like Dave Summers, the reporter at NBC 7, who for 34 years has covered the gamut of daily life, the good, bad and ugly.

All television news stations have "go-to" reporters and producers when all hell is breaking loose. "I'm the picture that you see when it says, "In Case of Emergency Break Glass," he jokes.

When asked whether he was concerned about his safety while covering the events of this time, he said, "I mean you always got your head on a swivel.... Did I fear for my life? Did I fear possible injury? Absolutely."

He recalled walking with 500 to 1,000 Black Lives Matter protesters through the middle of the street.

"I can't stand a block away, you've got to walk with them" for "understanding the emotion and the sense of what this is all about," he said. "Even in large groups there were subgroups that didn't really seem interested in making Black Lives Matter but were more interested in mayhem and breaking things."

"These drifters, these hangers," Summers called them, would take control after the group members "who seem sincere about making life better for Black people, about changing the culture and police, would go home."

Then came the confrontations with the police, swearing, and crossing police lines to create chaos.

"You felt bad for the folks and leadership of the group, the Black Lives Matter group, because it made them look violent and in the wrong," he said.

Summers was in La Mesa covering the confrontations between protestors, police and patriot groups. He was trapped between the groups and was "afraid of the police, not because they were bad, but because they have a job to do" but he was in the middle, catching it from all sides.

"We're media, we're going to be in the way," he acknowledged.

Avitia described the La Mesa riots as an ignition point for a growing number of people taking to the streets, driven by social media. The actual physical scene had angry, frustrated people lashing out, he said.

"There were these conflicts, tensions between business owners, the protesters, then you had city officials, and policemen. So there's these different factions that are really, you know, they're not cooperating, they're not talking to each other, everything's kind of radicalized, and everyone's in their own corner. I can tell you that predominantly White men were perpetuating violence during that day."

Rasahanna Lee and her partner helped organize one protest in La Mesa. She said she was chilled when she saw the large police contingent.

"You would think they were going to Iraq," she recalled.

Eventually, she said, "we were on our knees, looking at the police with thousands of dollars of gear on, and we are unarmed protestors, our only defense was pleading, 'don't shoot us.'"

It was a frightening experience that gave her a feeling of helplessness, she said. "There was nothing you could say or do."

She and her partner helped organize the protest, and she recalls, "I was a target, after this I don't see how anyone could not get involved." Lee noted, "White women were as aggressive, if not more so, than their men; they had a role to play as Trump supporters."

Summers said, "We saw patriot groups that were standing on the perimeter of a Black Lives Matter march that was in front of the police station."

Working the sidelines in La Mesa was an active blogger and organizer of hate group gatherings, Roger Ogden. Ogden is a well-known figure in hate group circles and familiar to Binkowski who tracks hate groups. Ogden, Binkowski alleges, is a disciple of David Duke, the Klansman, and Tom Metzger. Binkowski said it is no surprise that Ogden is active in border and immigration policies and politics. He has a blog called

Patriot Fire where "[h]e gets people to do things for him, he incites violence everywhere," Binkowski claims.

Summers recalled Ogden's appearances at the protests he covered, saying, "[T]hat guy shows up everywhere I show up."

Ogden's efforts were widely reported in 2017, when he was the organizer of two "patriot picnics" at Chicano Park. He claimed their only intention was to have a peaceful picnic in the park to prove "real patriot Americans" weren't allowed in the park. As one might imagine, this turned chaotic, and Ogden was seen with various White supremacy groups who were in attendance.

Videos, still photos, social media posts and local news accounts have shown Ogden active in his support of the Proud Boys and other White nationalist organizations that identify as Trump supporters. His blog, "Patriot Fire, "contains various descriptions of White supremacists' actions in the region and nationally. I attempted to speak with Ogden regarding his perspective, but he never responded to numerous efforts.

The trail to find how the local action related to the larger picture happening across America began for me in a message with details from the first anti-vaxxer protest in downtown San Diego. It read:

> The crowd was large, mostly Trump supporters and they were filming us and the police.
>
> The organizer's name is Naomi Israel. She posted a flier on her Facebook page and I believe she is a member of the anti-vaccination movement. She never responded to my interview requests, and I couldn't find her Saturday. The protest was billed as a "Freedom Rally."

Protest organizer Naomi Israel quickly made a name for herself at the early protests. Also known as Naomi Soria, she organized at least two protests and was the first person charged by SDPD for a misdemeanor at an April rally in downtown San Diego. She would later brag on Facebook, "My protest made the frontpage."

Soria had been in communication previously with, according to stories in various media outlets, the Center for American Liberty out of the Bay Area run by Attorney Harmeet Dhillon. Dhillon, it was found, is close to former President Trump, speaking on his behalf on a variety of issues. She is the former vice chairwoman of the California Republican Party, and a National Committeewoman for the Republican National Committee for California. Some might find it curious that this close ally of Donald Trump would be handling a misdemeanor case in San Diego. Dhillon, for her part, was quoted in a story by NBC 7 saying she's "gone to bat in court for people of every political persuasion." During this period of unrest, she appeared regularly on Fox Cable News, joining Tucker Carlson and other Fox 'celebrities' in advocating for the Trump agenda.

Numerous anti-vaxxers appeared to be driven by a mixed agenda of what they saw as patriotic duty to defend their rights and protect their health.

In Binkowski's opinion, "It's a lot of yoga-mom types who are roped in by anti-vaxxer bullshit."

These protestors adopted, as other alt-right groups would do, the American Flag as their symbol, wrapping themselves in the flag and characterizing anyone on the streets opposing them as traitors and anti-American. She says the anti-vax, anti-immigrant, anti-Black justice groups used the nation's flag as their symbol, to claim their interpretation of the American Constitution as what the Founding Fathers had intended.

Black Panther Wallace says he's been here before, seeing conflicts erupting on the streets of America and warns "we have a fragile democracy right now."

For him the protests of that winter and spring were a call to arms for Americans, no matter their race.

"People need to stay vigilant longer, we stay vigilant and stay involved in the political process and demand change, then this country will go forward on those on they're sitting on the fence, need to get off the fence and start realizing that if they don't become active, they won't save America."

Paul Krueger
Alejandra Sotelo-Solis—The Mayor of National City Takes On COVID-19

Less than two years on the job as the first Latina mayor of National City, Alejandra Sotelo-Solis confronted what would quickly consume her political time and energy. As the top elected official in a city with a huge Hispanic/Latino population (63.5 percent) and sizable Asian population (18.5 percent), Sotelo-Solis knew that outreach on the ground and at the workplace was the key to controlling the COVID-19 pandemic.

Another challenge: A big percentage of National City's 61,000 residents are "essential workers": health and home care aides; government employees; restaurant, supermarket and retail workers; and others at high risk for infection.

"These are people who can't work from home," Sotelo-Solis told me in December 2020. At that time, she was frustrated by the frequently changing government guidelines for masking and COVID-19 protection. "They are fatigued by all the changes," she said. "What's open and what's not? What do the different colored tiers [signifying infection rates] mean? They are fatigued by all these [constant] changes."

Her solution? "We need to be nimble and flexible in our response [to protect these people], but it's hard when the messages keep changing. It's frustrating." Yard signs were an obvious and convenient method for spreading basic, accurate information: "Cover Your Mouth!" "Keep Your Distance."

Sotelo-Solis found another strategy that worked: breaking down public health guidelines into easily understood "bite-sized pieces" or bullet points, that explain what her constituents should—and should not—do to avoid contracting that potentially life-threatening illness.

She applauded the County of San Diego for funding social service agencies that were already established in her community, so-called "trusted vessels," a term I also heard frequently in my COVID conversations with other Black and Brown community leaders. In National City, one important "trusted vessel" is the Latino Health Coalition, which Sotelo-Solis credits for helping "amplify" essential and accurate information about the virus and distributing 800 COVID-19 care packages, each with a face mask, thermometer, hand sanitizer, and easy-to-read information about the virus.

Sotelo-Solis correctly predicted that the county health department's vaccine campaign would face push-back from skeptics in her community. So she used her own credibility as Mayor to help persuade residents to roll up their arms. The mayor immediately enrolled in a UCSD COVID-19 vaccine trial and publicized her early decision to get vaccinated. "I asked [UCSD] staff if my personal involvement impacted participation in the [vaccine] trial," she told me. "They said traffic on their website had increased 150 percent, which was anecdotal evidence that my involvement in that trial helped build [community] trust."

The Mayor also learned that it's crucially important to stay ahead of misinformation about vaccine safety. "We have to have conversations about what the vaccine is [and isn't]. We need to have that dialogue with our [community] elders and dispel the myths. We have to describe in detail what the vaccine is and what it does." That means effectively communicating the most basic information, including that the vaccine is a shot, not a pill, and that it's given in either one or two doses, depending on the manufacturer.

In mid-December, the Mayor told me approximately 40 percent of her community had been vaccinated, a lower rate than she'd hoped for, and which she attributed to the lack of readily available information about the vaccine, its safety, and its ability to prevent infection.

When I checked back with Sotelo-Solis two weeks later, she was upbeat about the public education effort. She talked glowingly of a vaccination program at Paradise Valley Hospital, focused on the janitorial and maintenance crews, many of whom are people of color. "We highlighted a local [female employee], and all of her colleagues saw she was a Latina willing to step up and do what's needed for the greater good," by getting vaccinated.

"I was crying when I heard her story," the Mayor told me. "It felt so real." Sotelo-Solis wished more of the local media had covered that story. "There needs to be more images of front-line workers [getting their shots], not just doctors and medical professionals. She was also frustrated at the pace of the vaccine roll-out, which seemed to be in a "holding pattern" with indecision about "what's next, and who gets the vaccine."

She was sure that the key to boosting vaccine rates was to keep warning front-line, blue-collar workers about the long-term consequences of contracting the virus, including problems with lung and brain function. She also noted that many South Bay residents enlist in the military after high school and should know that that career path could be closed off to them if the long-term effects of COVID-19 made them ineligible for military service.

The Mayor said the pandemic has shined new light on existing healthcare inequities in our lower-income neighborhoods, including higher rates of diabetes, obesity, and other often-preventable diseases that can cause serious complications for COVID-19 patients. "The Biden administration does now understand the need for resources [that help our community] know who to call, how to get a translator, and how to make an appointment for routine care, which is [often] not a problem if you're an English-speaker."

Even as vaccination rates continued to climb in 2021, Sotelo-Solis highlighted the long-term positives. "This pandemic has offered us so many opportunities to partner with social service agencies, and there are now real opportunities to improve [everything from] health care to food distribution," she told me.

Though the Delta variant was putting thousands of unvaccinated (and a few vaccinated) San Diegans in the ICU in the summer of 2021, the Mayor reflected on what were, for her, the lessons learned from the pandemic.

On a personal level, Sotelo-Solis said she was "most proud of participating in the COVID-19 vaccine trial for Johnson & Johnson and sharing my experience publicly, and on-camera...sharing tests [results], nasal swabs, blood draws, and updates on my daily symptoms with my community via social media [to help] dispel vaccine myths and help inform my community of the benefits of being vaccinated."

In hindsight, Sotelo-Solis said she wishes "we had more resources at the onset of the pandemic to help people and youth with mental health resources on how to cope with COVID-19 fears, anxieties, and potential long-term health impacts."

On a positive note, the Mayor congratulated the medical community for "providing timely medical information both in person and via social media, [providing] volunteers for vaccination efforts, and helping us access personal protection equipment for our region." Sotelo-Solis said it's important to keep tabs on the community's needs moving forward, to better provide support and assets for the community.

Regarding the role of local, state, and federal governments in the continuing effort to vaccine against COVID-19 and the Delta variant, the Mayor highlighted the importance of funding for "community-driven efforts that are proving successful, and not count it as a victory until we reach the 75 percent vaccination rate in all communities, especially those hardest hit by COVID-19-positive rates, and its economic impact and death rates."

Paul Krueger
Forging Trust—The Pandemic and San Diego's Black Community

Wendy Shurelds eventually changed her mind about the COVID-19 vaccine, but not for the reasons you might assume.

Wendy is a veteran community health organizer, breast cancer survivor, and founder of "Many Shades of Pink," an advocacy and education effort that helps spread the word in San Diego's Black community about breast cancer detection and treatment.

Wendy's extensive discussions with community members has exposed her to the deeply-rooted skepticism and distrust of the mostly-White medical establishment. She's heard—and empathizes with—the talk about Black lives needlessly lost to the Tuskegee syphilis "experiments," and the concerns that Black communities have historically either been deprived of adequate medical care, or worse, used as "guinea pigs" for unproven treatments.

"I'm a Black woman, and I've worked in the medical field for 25 years," Wendy told me. "I've seen lots of things I shouldn't have seen. I've seen lots of Black patients who didn't receive the same type of [quality medical] treatment, not even basic treatment, as our White counterparts were offered. I do believe that medical professionals have biases. It's just within them, and it will show."

Wendy's personal experience with those racial disparities—and her familiarity with the extensive clinical trials usually required for FDA approval of new medications and medical treatments—were the basis of her deep skepticism that the COVID-19 vaccines had, in fact, been adequately tested.

When we first talked in late 2020, as news of the imminent availability of the vaccines dominated the headlines, Wendy was also very concerned that there wasn't enough information available on the vaccines' possible side effects, given the rush to develop those preventative treatments. "I feel like they just don't have enough short- or long-term data," she explained. "It's a really big deal for me. Sometimes, even with a lot of data, we don't learn until years later that even [treatments] with FDA approval can cause other diseases."

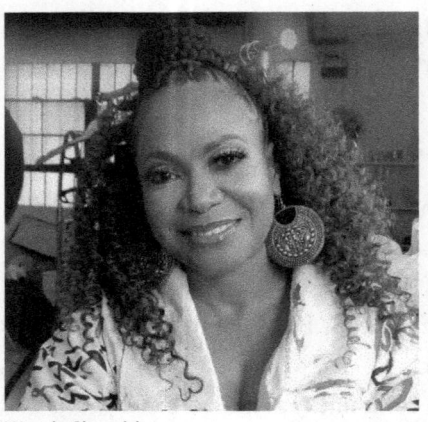
Wendy Shurelds

Wendy told me her sentiments were shared by many of her friends, with whom she chatted on Facebook. And her own skepticism about vaccine safety made it easy for her to understand why many others in San Diego's Black community would "take the risk of getting COVID-19 instead of getting the vaccine."

She acknowledged that the importance of quickly developing an effective vaccine had prompted an unprecedented and vigorous research and testing effort that by all appearances did not shortcut safety protocols. She also acknowledged that the science behind the vaccines and the safety data to date was impressive. But she remained deeply skeptical. "No," Wendy told me. "I'm not buying it. Even if [Dr. Anthony] Fauci called me personally, I'm not taking [the vaccine]. Even when Fauci says one of his top scientists is a Black woman, that's not enough.

Wendy had another, very reasonable rationale for shunning the vaccine. She was confident that her personal safety protocols put her at a very low risk for contracting the virus. She was not an essential worker, she diligently followed all safety protocols, and rarely even left her home. Taking those precautions made her confident she would not be exposed to the virus.

Wendy's tough stance and strong opinions set me up for a big surprise when we talked again on January 31, 2021.

By then, the vaccines were widely available, and San Diegans lined up by the thousands to get "the shot." And, much to my surprise, Wendy was one of them.

"I got the vaccine," she told me. Though her "mind was so made up that no one could change it," she relented, for two reasons.

First, she had decided to work at a public community health and resource fair and didn't want to risk being exposed to the virus.

Second, and more important, was the birth of her first grandchild. "I wanted to see my grandson," Wendy explained.

Her skepticism about the thoroughness of the vaccine trials and her fear of side effects was also tempered by a series of webinars she had watched, at least one of which featured Dr. Rodney Hood, a long-time leader in San Diego's Black medical community.

"I educated myself on the things I had issues with," Wendy told me. "In some areas, I was not informed."

For example, Wendy told me she had thought the vaccines contained a "live virus," which had deeply concerned her. She later learned that none of the vaccines have the "live virus" and that they were developed in a manner that satisfied her safety concerns. She also took a second, much closer look at the vaccines' safety data. "Before, I felt like there was not enough time spent on studying the side effects, but I saw they were very minimal. So I was like, 'Okay, I'm very happy with that.'"

She also saw a presentation by a panel of Black physicians, who reassured their audience that "this is not a vaccine that is out to harm Black people or people of color." Those reassurances resonated with her because they were spoken by "someone who looks like me, who understands my fears and my concerns, and who can relate to what I'm concerned about." Wendy acknowledged that White doctors can also understand her concerns, but she thinks they are unable to "fully understand the trauma that a certain race has been through because of racial disparities [in healthcare]."

Once she was convinced of the vaccines' safety and got the shots, she spread the word on her Facebook page and the Facebook page for her "Many Shades of Pink" breast cancer awareness group. "There are so many people who, bottom line, just don't get it. They're concerned that doctors are trying to put some sort of tracking device in us. They have so many myths and conspiracies on this."

Her advice to the Black community: "Educate yourself. Get knowledge. Don't close your mind and [think] you're not going to get the virus." Instead, she wanted everyone to know what she told her uncle: "You can get the vaccine, or you can get COVID."

And when we chatted again about COVID and vaccine skepticism, Wendy told me her efforts had persuaded at least one skeptic to get vaccinated: the day after she had talked with her uncle, he had agreed to get "the shot."

Paul Krueger
Meet People Where They Are

With the county in the grips of the first of several deadly surges in the COVID-19 pandemic, Dr. Suzanne Afflalo told me the biggest failing by health officials was their inability "to meet the people where they are."

Afflalo, an African American, is a local community health physician who is well-qualified to critique the government's response to the pandemic. "The county health department has done a good job of general messaging [about the danger of COVID-19]," she told me. "But we need to get 'trusted messengers' into the [BIPOC] community, at the churches, and other places where the people are."

Meeting community members face-to-face where they live, work, worship, and play was the key to combating misinformation about both the virus, and the vaccine (which hadn't been rolled out when we first talked). "We had mixed messages from the beginning," Dr. Afflalo explained, "and we should have gotten in front of this, gotten out there sooner. We needed to tell people to stay off social media, and work to debunk the myths."

Dr. Afflalo said mistrust of the nation's medical establishment among Blacks and widespread misinformation when the virus first appeared made "a bad situation 50 times worse." She cites, for example, a rumor that started early on to the effect that "Black people can't get the virus. It targets only older, White people."

Another falsehood, spread by word-of-mouth and social media, was that there was "one vaccine for White people and another for Blacks, which will make you sterile."

Dr. Afflalo told me those sorts of wild rumors—amplified by social media—caused some people of color to "just go about their business" and ignore masking and social distancing. "We're playing catch-up the whole time," she said when we first talked.

To combat this misinformation, Black healthcare and community workers held a series of community forums in which "trusted messengers" from the community talked about COVID-19's real threat. They stressed the fact that, according to Dr. Afflalo, "Blacks have a much, much higher death rate" from COVID, due in part to higher rates of diabetes, asthma, and other co-morbidities. "We needed to tell them, bluntly, that if they want to be around next Thanksgiving and next Christmas, and if they want to see your loved ones, they need to get that vaccine.'"

Her efforts—and those of other dedicated health care and social service providers—were made even more difficult when Shane Harris grabbed the local media's attention in late December 2020. Harris is an outspoken young Black man whose tenacity and ability to command news coverage often puts him in front of the camera on hot-button issues, including police-community relations and cases of alleged racial discrimination.

This time, Harris generated coverage with his controversial statement that he would not get the Pfizer vaccine (or, apparently, any other vaccine), and would not encourage any community members to get vaccinated.

"He has a megaphone,' Dr. Afflalo said, acknowledging Harris's influence. She moved quickly to rebut Harris's statement and limit its damage. She told me she called Harris and told him—clearly and concisely: "The way you're delivering that information is making our job harder. You have already tainted our effort by giving incorrect information."

She told me Harris listened respectfully and acknowledged that he hadn't "packaged his message well."

Dr. Afflalo also expressed frustration that the medical community's outreach efforts weren't working as hoped and that county government officials and community leaders were spending too much time on "Zoom meetings, where we were just speaking to the choir."

Eventually, Dr. Afflalo's message—amplified by other Black health care providers—did spread. By early 2021, she was guardedly optimistic that outreach efforts were working, thanks in part to work done by the county's public health department and its director, Dr. Wilma Wooten. "We're working with the pastors [at local Black churches], we're educating a handful of the 'trusted messengers' who can debunk the myths and promote the vaccine," Dr. Afflalo told me. "We're trying to plant the seeds, and get more people involved, so they know the facts, understand the science, and can refute the myths."

But the audience for those "trusted messengers" was overwhelmingly the older, church-going members of the Black community. The challenge remained: how to reach a younger generation that "isn't within the four walls [of a church or social group) as much?"

That required more outreach to younger community leaders, who can hold their generation's attention.

There also remained unique challenges in persuading Black community members—young and old—to get the vaccine, including the real and shameful legacy of the Tuskegee syphilis experiments, in which hundreds of Black men were denied available and effective treatment for that potential deadly disease.

As the second wave of COVID infections started to subside in October 2021, Dr. Afflalo told me that Black San Diegans, especially in the 18-39–year age group, continued to have "reservations and concerns" about the vaccines, despite all the medical evidence of their life-saving effectiveness.

"Social media, which is the dominant source of information for most young adults, is filled with misinformation and disinformation about

COVID-19," she lamented. "The younger population believe they don't need to get vaccinated because they are healthy, without any underlying health conditions, so they feel they won't get severely ill if they do get infected by COVID-19." Of course, nothing could be further from the truth, with a pandemic that has killed and critically injured tens of thousands of San Diegans, without regard to race, color, creed, class status, sex, or age.

As the impact of the Delta variant waned in the fall of 2021, Dr. Afflalo reflected on the impediments to wider vaccination among our Black residents. She told me that the county health department was never able to clearly determine which of our ethnic communities were being impacted the most by the pandemic and lamented yet again the late start that public health offices got in countering vaccine skepticism. "So misinformation, disinformation, and myths became rooted in various communities of color, thus making it extremely difficult to undo the damage that had already been done," Dr. Afflalo said.

She also noted that vaccine distribution was "not equitable" during the crucial early months, so fewer people of color, "who represent a disproportionate amount of the [county's] vulnerable essential and frontline workers, were unable to get the vaccine."

Getting an appointment for the vaccine when it first became available was, of course, a challenge for many San Diegans, regardless of their color or income level. But Dr. Afflalo says getting the shot was "nearly impossible for people of color," who she said face significant additional challenges, including their inability to leave their jobs mid-shift, the initial unavailability of evening hours at vaccine clinics, limited transportation to distant vaccine sites, and a lack of internet and computer access for scheduling.

But Dr. Afflalo did praise state and local health officials for strictly limiting public events to control the initial virus, making virus testing widely available, and imposing a vaccine mandate for health care workers, teachers and school staff, and students aged 12-18.

One of the biggest lessons learned—and one that she says can best serve our community if COVID-19 surges again, or another pandemic surfaces—is the crucial role of community-based organizations in spreading the word about safe practices and proper response. "I think our community-based organizations did a better job of educating the BIPOC community than government could have done," she concluded. "That's why it was wise for state and local governments to partner with—and fund—the organizations to do that work. It was necessary to get those 'trusted messengers' to reach the BIPOC communities."

Gabriella Rodriguez
COVID-19: The Most Powerful Border Wall Ever, A Binational Economic Killer

When the pandemic first started and California Governor Gavin Newsom ordered non-essential workers to stay home, Amanda, a Mexican national, was in North Park, a neighborhood of San Diego, California. She was on the job taking care of a then 3-year-old toddler she had been a nanny to since the child was only 4 months old. "As I started to see people losing their jobs, I was just grateful I still had mine," explained Amanda.

Her job as a childcare provider was deemed essential; however, her home was in Tijuana. She usually crossed the border to come to work once a week, with her tourist visa. "I lived with the family I worked for during the week and returned to my home in Tijuana over the weekend to spend time with my daughter. It was tough being away from her for many days, but it was a sacrifice I was willing to make so I could help her achieve her dreams of going to law school one day," Amanda explained.

Things took a complex turn when the Trump administration announced it would close the U.S./Mexico border to nonessential travel; among things deemed nonessential was tourism. Amanda was faced with making a tough decision. She would either go home to Tijuana jobless and likely not be able to find a job mid-pandemic or stay in the U.S. and ride out the pandemic with the family she worked for.

In hopes the border would eventually reopen once things were under control, Amanda decided to stay in the U.S. "I thought, there is no way they will keep the border closed to tourists for too long. San Diego and

Tijuana stimulate each other's economy." One of the most gut-wrenching parts of Amanda's decision was not being able to see her 17-year-old daughter and leaving her alone to fend for herself in the middle of a global pandemic.

As the pandemic continued to take over the world and eventually California, the likelihood of the border reopening seemed like less of a possibility. "With every month that passed, I worried that there was no end in sight. I worried about my daughter. Who would take care of her if she was exposed to the virus?" said Amanda. The conditions in Tijuana were getting worse each day. Hospitals were overrun; doctors and medical staff were being forced to buy PPE with their own money.

After 8 months of not being able to return home and the holidays approaching, Amanda decided to return home to be with her daughter during the holidays. "I just couldn't leave her alone for the holidays. I needed the job and the money, but I am a mother first, and I knew I would find a way to make it work. I had to," Amanda says about her decision to return to Mexico.

"The joy of being around my daughter after so many months was worth it," explains Amanda. Both mother and daughter took the time to enjoy the holidays together and catch up after so many months of being apart, but in just a few weeks Amanda was forced to get creative to make an income. She started a side hustle selling food. This type of work increased her exposure to people. Within just a month of being back, Amanda and her daughter both got infected with the virus. Luckily her daughter had mild symptoms, but Amanda was bedridden for weeks. Amanda's only chance at getting medical attention was the public healthcare system, the same place where doctors were quitting because they didn't have PPE and were afraid of dying from the virus or giving it to their families.

"During the pandemic, people often said we are all on the same boat, but that couldn't be further from the truth. We may all be in the same turbulent waters, but some of us are in yachts while others are in the water without a life vest just trying to stay above water," Amanda said.

Will Huntsberry, Jesse Marx, and Bella Ross

The First Year of COVID: A College Degree Was an "Insurance Policy" Against Death

This story was first published by Voice of San Diego with support from the Fund for Investigative Journalism.

November 30, 2021

Gregory Denny didn't get his bachelor's degree until he was 48 years old—and not until after his death from COVID-19.

Denny, a veteran, was a security specialist at Taylor Guitars in El Cajon. He'd been doing private security work since coming home from the Gulf War in the early '90s. He got married and raised two children.

But when he hit his 40s, Denny was struck with a burst of middle-aged aspiration. He decided to get a bachelor's degree and by June 2020 was only a few weeks away from completion. That's when he caught the novel coronavirus, which took his life on July 24, 2020.

In honor of his work and life, American Military University in Virginia posthumously awarded him with a bachelor's degree, making him a member of the graduating class of 2021.

Denny's story exemplifies a cruel truth about the pandemic: That having a bachelor's degree and the elevated job status that comes with it often marked the distance between life and death.

Income and education levels have already been linked with increased risk of death among COVID-19 patients. But a new Voice of San Diego analysis shows, in disturbing detail, how the pandemic disproportionately killed San Diegans with lower levels of education and income.

Voice of San Diego reviewed 4,046 death certificates, one for each COVID-related death in San Diego County beginning with the first on March 22, 2020, and ending a year later.

Only 17 percent of people who died in San Diego County had a bachelor's degree or higher. But 40 percent of people 25 and older have that same level of education countywide, according to U.S. Census Bureau data. Another 31 percent of victims didn't have a high school diploma, which is also significantly out of line with countywide figures.

"In many ways, the presence of having a bachelor's degree for individuals during the pandemic was really an insurance policy," said Audrey Dow, senior vice president of the Campaign for College Opportunity, a public advocacy and research group. "It was really a prevention asset."

Having a bachelor's degree is often the distinguishing factor between essential workers and those who worked from home during the pandemic.

Denny, for instance, was still working in-person at Taylor Guitars when he contracted COVID-19. That's where his wife, Kimberly, thinks he got it, though she doesn't blame the company.

People like Denny had to be physically present at their place of employment, while many with a college education were at home, designing personal office spaces and learning how to use Zoom.

After Denny's death, Kimberly didn't leave their house in Jamul for a long time. Her life was thrown off its course. But it was Denny's memory that forced her back outside.

"Greg wouldn't want me sitting in my house," she said. "He wouldn't want us to be crying for sure."

She sold the house and moved to Arizona.

The American Dream cannot reconcile itself to the idea that outcomes of any kind—like the job a person has or the age at which they die—are determined by a person's ZIP code and not their character. But the analysis of local death certificates makes clear that COVID-19 traveled along the socioeconomic fault lines of San Diego and made them even wider.

Pandemic deaths by ZIP code, class, or education level all tell the same story: San Diegans with less died more.

"Those factors are significantly more influential in terms of our health status than things like our inherent biology or even healthcare," said Tyan Parker Dominguez, University of Southern California clinical professor and chair of the School of Social Work.

Where you live and the job you do, in other words, has more impact on your health than your own DNA or access to healthcare. As a logical proposition, it hardly seems to make sense. The reasons are many, and may seem small on their own, but together create a wall that is nearly impossible for poverty to pass through.

Take, for instance, food deserts. It's well documented that poorer neighborhoods have few or no grocery stores. They are much more likely to have a Family Dollar and a drive-thru window.

"It's very costly to eat healthy food. It costs less to eat off the McDonald's menu," said Maria Rosario Araneta, a professor of public health at UC San Diego.

But eating off the fast-food menu clogs arteries and elevates sugars. It leads to chronic health conditions like diabetes and heart disease, which make you far more likely to die from COVID. Out of the 4,000-plus deaths analyzed by Voice of San Diego, approximately 80 percent of people were suffering from a chronic health condition. Of those, 25 percent had diabetes.

ZIP code 92113, which stretches from Barrio Logan to Lincoln Park, had one of the highest death rates in the entire county. And it has some of the fewest options for buying healthy food and produce, said Araneta.

"There's no Vons, no Sprouts, no Trader Joe's and there's definitely not a Whole Foods," she said.

It's not just food deserts that make working-class people more susceptible to chronic disease, though. Poorer adolescents literally have higher blood pressure than their peers. Blood pressure above a certain point is considered hypertension, which is also more common among people with lower incomes. Hypertension increases the likelihood of strokes and heart attacks and was also a common condition listed on the COVID death certificates.

The stress that comes with poverty, in other words, increases a person's health risks.

And consider the many risks, the many incidental hazards. Poor people were more likely to need public transportation during COVID, making them more exposed. They were more likely to live in cramped or precarious housing—with people who were more likely to be going out into the world every day as essential workers, in grocery stores, retail stores, and old people's homes.

The lower someone slides on society's ladder, the more these risks close in around them.

As part of the analysis, Voice logged nearly all the information contained on each death certificate into a database. An occupation was listed for each individual, as well as educational attainment and other data points. Voice then grouped each job into categories that align with U.S. Census Bureau definitions.

The analysis suggests COVID disproportionately killed working-class San Diegans.

The most frequently listed occupation was "homemaker." Those made up 15 percent of all deaths.

The median age of death was 76—which may explain why homemakers made up such a large percentage of those who died. Women of older generations were more likely to stay out of the workforce.

Out of the 10 most frequently listed job categories, excluding homemakers, only two have a median income of more than $50,000 a year.

The largest category is somewhat all-encompassing for entry-level jobs. It includes administration, support services, and waste management. Secretaries, custodians, security guards, and landscapers all fit into this category.

Construction workers, who remained "essential" throughout the pandemic and even experienced an increase in demand in 2020, made up the second largest class of occupations.

"Those who don't have a bachelor's degree or a high school degree are more likely to work in manual activities, customer service, agriculture, manufacturing, and other economic activities that don't allow them to stay safely at home," said Arturo Bustamante, a UCLA public health associate professor.

Three out of every four people who died during the first year of the pandemic were older than 65. Most of them were likely retired, even if they had an occupation listed on their death certificate. In that sense, the occupations listed are a more accurate reflection of a person's class than whether they performed essential work during the pandemic.

Even still, more than 1,000 working age people died—and many of them performed essential labor.

Francisco Rubio, like Denny, worked in private security.

Francisco, like many of those who died, had a health condition that made him more vulnerable to the novel coronavirus. He struggled with obesity and was in and out of the hospital due to infections and blood clots. When he was younger, his family moved from unincorporated East County to San Diego so he could be closer to medical professionals.

Jackie Rubio remembered her son as a funny and lovable guy who did impressions and might have been a comedian. He also loved cars—"that was his joy," she said—and before testing positive for COVID-19 in December 2020 he'd been making plans to study automotive repair.

The family was on the way to the hospital on New Year's Day to say their goodbyes when Francisco passed away. He was 21.

Though obesity put Francisco at risk and made it harder for his body to fight back, COVID-19 was considered the primary cause of death. COVID-19, however, was not listed as the primary cause in each of the death certificates Voice examined. In 7 percent of cases it was listed as a contributing cause, rather than a primary cause.

A comparison of median household income and death rates shows a clear statistical relationship between the two. Higher income ZIP codes had lower death rates, and vice-versa.

In fact, for every $6,600 increase in household income, the rate of death went down by 10 percent, said David Meyer, a mathematics professor at UCSD, who reviewed Voice's data.

A Carmel Valley ZIP code, 92130, ranked first in household income and also had the lowest death rate, at 0.3 deaths per every 1,000 residents. A San Ysidro ZIP code, 92173, had one of the lowest median incomes and the highest death rate, at 3.4 deaths per every 1,000 residents.

Race and ethnicity are also inextricably linked with income in the United States. Roughly 55 percent of the residents who live in the Carmel Valley ZIP code identify as White-only, for instance. More than 90 percent of the people living in the San Ysidro ZIP code identify as Latino.

On the whole, Whites and Latinos experienced opposite effects during the pandemic. San Diego County residents who identify as White-only accounted for 33 percent of deaths during the first year of the pandemic, while accounting for 43 percent of residents. Latinos represent roughly 34 percent of county residents, but 47 percent of deaths in the first year of the pandemic.

"People with less income, and Black and brown folks, are the folks who are going to be at higher risk, historically, for adverse health outcomes," Dominguez said.

The facts of COVID are indisputable: Latinos died more often; the less educated died more often; and poor people died more often. What's up for debate is why.

Some believe, with research to support them, that vulnerable citizens face death by a thousand cuts. The public and private institutions of the country—everything from grocery stores to governments—are contaminated with racial and class inequality, the thinking goes.

But a whole other swath of people doesn't believe that at all. They believe the United States gives you back whatever you deserve.

It's a colossal disagreement. But focusing on the facts we know could still empower better decision-making in the future, according to public health experts.

"Knowing this information about who are the high-risk groups could have certainly guided policies, decisions around resource allocation, and around thinking about targeted strategies for ameliorating risk and the spread of disease," said Dominguez.

One of those early strategies was COVID-19 testing. And testing centers were not located in the most vulnerable areas of San Diego in the earliest days, said Araneta, the public health professor at UCSD.

In other words, officials put more testing centers in places where they were needed less.

Vaccination sites were also not clustered in places with the highest infection rates early on, Araneta said.

Many people would assume the United States has the greatest health care system in the world, that it is more prepared to weather disaster than any other nation, and the standard of living is unequaled. Some San Diegans do live in the safety of that America. But the massively unequal results brought about by the pandemic challenge those assumptions.

"It's another example of a disease that affects a broad swath of the population disproportionately," said Robert Schooley, an infectious disease specialist at UC San Diego Health, "one of the things that perpetuates our caste system of people who have means."

Brad Racino and Jill Castellano

Health Experts, Residents Worry South County Not Ready for Reopening As COVID-19 Worsens

> *This story was originally produced and published by inewsource, a nonprofit, nonpartisan newsroom in San Diego committed to exposing wrongdoing and holding powerful people and institutions accountable. As part of their commitment to keeping the San Diego community informed, inewsource has allowed this story to be reprinted and shared here with you. To learn more about their work and how you can support their journalism, visit inewsource.org.*

May 11, 2020

Inside the Sharp Chula Vista Medical Center on a recent Friday, nurse Richard Harchfield passed medical supplies through a sliding glass door. His colleagues in the isolation room were performing a battery of tests on a suspected COVID-19 patient while medical staff elsewhere in the hospital fought to keep alive 58 people stricken by the virus.

Upstairs, in the intensive care unit, doctors donned self-powered respirators to check on patients: One was strapped to a gurney that rotated to improve aeration in the lungs; another lay hooked up to a ventilator, sedated, with a small TV displaying a tranquil forest scene in a room no family members could visit.

Asked when COVID-19 cases peaked at the Sharp hospital, infection preventionist Cindy Stuart responded, "I feel like it's happening right now."

About a dozen miles north, outside the San Diego Hall of Justice that same Friday, hundreds of protesters gathered to urge Governor Gavin Newsom to reopen the state. Signs read, "All Jobs are Essential" and "COVID-19 Socialism Unleashed." A local radio host rallied the crowd with a bullhorn. A spa owner warned Newsom not to get a haircut once salons are allowed to operate again.

Scenes like those at Sharp and in downtown San Diego are playing out across the state and the country, where solutions for the economic devastation wrought by stay-at-home orders compete with the cautious approach urged by healthcare providers who want to save as many lives as they can.

Over the past several weeks, inewsource has interviewed San Diegans directly affected by COVID-19 to piece together a comprehensive picture of the harrowing tradeoff health officials must make: Appease struggling citizens who are pushing for a return to normal, or guard against an influx of cases in southern San Diego County that could devastate those communities.

This report was informed by time spent at the COVID-19 epicenter: the Sharp hospital caring for more coronavirus patients than anywhere else in the county. Reporters also spoke with a struggling small-business owner in San Marcos, a single mother in Imperial Beach unable to pay her rent, and a recovered COVID-19 patient from National City worried about his wife's health. They interviewed doctors, nurses, and hospital leaders trying to control hotspots in the South Bay.

Despite how the spread of the virus is unfolding in the South Bay, county officials decided on Friday it was time to ease restrictions on local businesses, allowing some non-essential stores to reopen for curbside pickup. When questioned about whether the decision could cause a spike in COVID-19 cases in South County, Public Health Officer Dr. Wilma Wooten said the region overall meets state and federal criteria to move forward.

"We have to look at the entire region, not just one area," Wooten said.

Taking Risks

At high-risk for developing COVID-19 complications, Patty Mendoza thinks it's too soon for the county to ease restrictions.

She earned just $400 in March with Ride Away, LLC, a non-emergency medical transport company, and was laid off in early April. Mendoza's 17-year-old daughter, her rock, reassured her the small family would make it work. Her 9-year-old son offered the money he earned from recycling cans and bottles toward their $1,500 monthly rent in Imperial Beach.

A single mother without a job, she said she cries in the shower where her two children won't see.

"I'm their mom. I'm supposed to be the strong one for them," Mendoza said through tears. "Sometimes I feel like I'm not. Sometimes now I feel like I'm failing."

Mendoza grew up in Tijuana and moved as a child with her parents to the South Bay.

In general, Hispanics like Mendoza are nearly three times as likely to test positive for COVID-19 as someone who is White, and more likely to test positive than African Americans and Asians, according to an inewsource analysis of county data. The analysis also found the infection rate for Hispanics in the county is increasing more quickly than it is for any other race or ethnicity.

Mendoza is also considered at a higher risk for developing a severe illness, like pneumonia, from COVID-19 because she has asthma, a condition that recently cost her a potential job at a grocery store.

She said the store manager worried frequent interactions with customers would put her at risk and explained, "I don't want to give you this job because what if you don't go back to your kids?"

The 44-year-old can't imagine getting to the point where she has to tell her kids they'll soon be homeless. She hasn't received her unemployment benefits or federal stimulus check yet, but she recently decided that getting a job would be too risky because of her health conditions and fears that in the coming weeks, with residents venturing out of their homes to parks or businesses, the risk will get higher.

"I think it's too soon. I think there's going to be another spike," Mendoza said.

Ailments like asthma, diabetes, and lung disease are clustered in the South County along with conditions that the U.S. Centers for Disease Control and Prevention says may affect that community's "ability to prevent human suffering and financial loss in the event of disaster." Those conditions include poverty, a lack of high school education, poor transportation options, single parent households, and high percentages of minorities. Combined, those factors determine an area's "social vulnerability" score, according to the CDC.

"We know that in disasters, the people on the margins of society are often the most impacted," said Corinne McDaniels-Davidson, director of the Institute for Public Health at San Diego State University.

"And what I mean by margins of society are those of limited means or low socioeconomic status—older adults and racial and ethnic minorities," she said.

McDaniels-Davidson pointed to the 1918 Spanish flu pandemic when the death rate from all causes among non-White populations was about 35% higher than among Whites. Jumping ahead to the 2009 H1N1 outbreak, she found "minority populations had about two-and-a-half to three-and-a-half times higher rates of hospitalization compared to non-Hispanic Whites."

The same day protesters gathered downtown and Sharp Chula Vista medical staff made the rounds, Mendoza and her children joined dozens of others in a rent protest that began with a caravan of cars outside a parking lot in San Ysidro and ended more than 20 miles north in Linda Vista.

Wearing a mask, Mendoza hung makeshift banners on her white Honda Odyssey minivan.

"The people's fight for a worthy life," read one in Spanish. "Governor Newsom Cancel Rent/Mortgage," said another.

"This is the story of my life right now," Mendoza said. "This is something that was not my fault."

"I didn't ask for this."

Opening the Door

Farther north, at the other end of the county, small-business owner Jeff McNeilly is also feeling the pinch—and he wants the county to let him reopen his shop.

By the time Newsom issued a stay-at-home order on March 19, McNeilly's Big Frog Custom T-Shirts & More store in San Marcos was barely hanging on.

Though he would celebrate the store's two-year anniversary in May, revenue was down around $20,000 in March, McNeilly said.

"Which is not a lot of money for many businesses, but for a small business like mine it's significant," he said.

McNeilly, who said he has burned through much of his savings just getting the business started, determined the state's order categorized his work as "non-essential." The 58-year-old felt his only choice was to close the store and move to online and phone orders.

"I have no idea what the future looks like," he said. "It's just hard to fathom at this point."

San Diego County's unemployment rate was estimated to be 27% at the end of April. A recent survey of local businesses found 75% plan to furlough or lay off employees, temporarily shut down operations, or permanently close.

McNeilly said we're not "all in this together," as people like to say.

"We might all be in the same storm, but we all have different pain, for sure."

Near the end of April, county Supervisor Jim Desmond, whose district includes North County, called for some businesses to reopen. He cited the economic toll of COVID-19 and the fact that businesses like Costco have proven their ability to handle thousands of customers safely. Mayors from Carlsbad, Escondido, Oceanside, San Marcos, and Vista joined him in urging the county to reopen businesses.

"We need to crack this door open. We need to start the economy going again," Desmond said.

It's not just closed businesses that have riled people.

Coronado Mayor Richard Bailey criticized county officials in a KUSI interview and op-ed in mid-April for closing off the oceans from recreational use.

He called the orders an abuse of power.

"The public deserves to be treated with trust and respect," he wrote. "Policies that are arbitrary, inconsistently applied, and criminalize harmless activities erode the public's trust."

By any metric, the county's stay-at-home mandates have stifled the virus's spread. A model developed by Dr. Natasha Martin, an infectious disease specialist at UC San Diego, estimates social distancing has saved 6,000 to 18,000 lives. Newsom lauded the county's handling of COVID-19.

County officials have cautioned against a rapid return to normal, warning that lifting restrictions too quickly because people are antsy could cause an unmanageable surge in cases like those experienced in Singapore over the past month.

Instead, they've said they are basing decisions on a series of metrics outlined by state and federal authorities that indicate how much control the region has over the virus. Every weekday, Wooten, the public health officer, presents those numbers at a news conference to keep residents up to date.

On May 1, Wooten said the county had successfully met four of the federal government's five criteria for reopening America, but added it's not performing enough COVID-19 tests to meet the fifth.

"These criteria must be met before states and regions can proceed with a phased approach to open up," she said.

Four days later, the fifth criterion still unfulfilled, Wooten announced the county would be ready to start lifting restrictions within the next few days.

"Based on available data, we feel we are ready," she said.

Wooten later explained that even though the region hadn't met the federal guidelines on testing, it had met the state's—conducting roughly 2,000 tests a day or more.

Under the new rules, which were created at the state level and recently enacted, some businesses—including bookstores, clothing stores, and sporting goods retailers—can reopen and offer curbside pickup to customers so long as they enforce social distancing and mask-wearing.

Wooten and others have emphasized that they are still watching COVID-19 metrics closely, and if they begin to see a surge in cases, they might shut down the businesses again.

McNeilly, the T-shirt store owner, said he believes he can open up safely by following the rules the county has laid out for essential businesses like grocery stores—sanitizing the shop, asking customers to stay six feet apart and making sure everyone wears face coverings.

"People online are like, 'If you want to open up the economy, that means you want people to die,'" he said. "The arguments are just so extreme, and that's not the case at all. I want to open up and do it safely."

Keeping businesses closed forever is not an option, McNeilly said.

"It's just not going to work. At some point I'm going to have to pay my bills, and I don't have the income to do it."

Flattening the Curve

Inside Sharp Chula Vista Medical Center, registered nurse, and infection preventionist Myra Laurino said she understands the frustration felt by McNeilly and others.

"There's so many people not working right now," and at some point we have to start the economy back up, she said.

"But we all want to do it in a safe manner, too."

Laurino walked through the hospital's ICU, which sounded like a wind tunnel as negative pressure ventilation ensured the virus didn't escape the dozens of rooms set up to house COVID-19 patients.

Nearby, Dr. Alejandro Villegas looked through the glass at a 75-year-old patient and smiled.

"Twenty-five days on a ventilator and we extubated him yesterday," Villegas said. "He's actually transitioning out of the ICU today."

One bright spot in an otherwise dark corner of San Diego County.

The hospitals Sharp and Scripps operate in Chula Vista have more COVID-19 patients than any other hospitals in the county, and the patients they test for the virus are more likely to test positive.

According to hospital officials interviewed in late April, Sharp Chula Vista was seeing roughly 20% of its patients test positive for COVID-19. At Scripps, the numbers ranged from 17% to 29%. Countywide, about 6% to 7% of tests come back positive each day.

What does that mean?

"Well, it means that we have an issue in the South County," said Chris Van Gorder, CEO of Scripps Health.

Projections that Scripps provided to inewsource show the unequal impact the virus has had throughout the county: In its La Jolla and Encinitas hospitals, the number of COVID-19 hospitalizations are expected to zero out starting in July. But in Chula Vista, if more mitigation efforts don't take place, the hospital anticipates a surge that will peak in September with about 300 COVID-19 patients at the same time.

Scripps has faced a continued growth in COVID-19 patients at its Chula Vista hospital over the past month and a recent spike in cases at its Mercy San Diego hospital in Hillcrest, where it's transferring patients to free needed beds in the South Bay.

Sharp has also begun transferring COVID-19 patients from its Chula Vista hospital to Sharp Memorial in Kearny Mesa and Sharp Grossmont in La Mesa—all to make room for the continuing influx of new coronavirus patients in the South Bay.

Hospital Safety Precautions

With some ill people not going to the hospital when they need emergency care out of fear of contracting COVID-19, Sharp officials wanted to assure the public safety measures are in place at its facilities. They said staff are putting significant distance between COVID-19 patients and the rest of the hospital population in addition to many other preventative measures.

Dan Gross, who retired last month as Sharp HealthCare's executive vice president but is continuing as a consultant, told inewsource he can't say for sure why hospitalizations are so much higher in South County, but the region's proximity to Mexico might be a factor.

"Tijuana is in crisis today," Gross said, "in terms of their hospitals, in terms of the number of positive COVID patients."

Gross and Van Gorder wrote a letter on April 28 to the U.S. Department of Health and Human Services about the situation.

"Any impression that we are flattening our curve ignores the threat south of the border," they said.

"Providers in the San Diego region do not have adequate supplies to meet the projections we anticipate as a result of the increasing cases in our border communities."

Scripps's case numbers show that more than a third of patients who have visited its Chula Vista hospital since the beginning of March had recently traveled to Mexico, though it couldn't determine where those patients contracted the virus. The day Van Gorder spoke with inewsource, he received a note from the county saying 11 ambulance runs had come from the border to county hospitals, and all of the patients were U.S. citizens.

But the hospital executives are struggling to make sense of the statistics coming out of Mexico. The Mexican government has been slow to test residents, so the number of COVID cases may appear lower than they actually are. It's also retroactively adding new COVID-19 positive tests to their data from people who contracted it days or weeks earlier, causing the numbers to change dramatically. Meanwhile, news stories reported a surge in cases at local hospitals that's expected to continue in the coming weeks.

"I know many people have questioned, 'What is the robustness and the accuracy of the data, and what is the strength of the infrastructure to truly capture all of the data under the current crises?" Gross said.

"That is indeed a question that is, I think, relevant and appropriate to be bringing forward," he said.

In late April, the county said hospitals could resume elective surgeries, such as tumor removal surgeries and repairing dislocated joints. Elective surgeries, which are more profitable to perform than emergency care is, were put on hold at the start of the pandemic to save room for COVID-19 patients.

Van Gorder said Scripps hospitals are starting to offer those procedures again but are doing it carefully and slowly so they don't use up too much protective medical gear and can watch out for a growth in COVID-19 cases—a growth he believes is inevitable once the county loosens restrictions.

"I think our elected officials must be under enormous pressure to reopen," Van Gorder said. "And I understand the impact on the economy. I mean Scripps, like every healthcare system, is losing money right now as well, but my responsibility is health-related, and I just want to make sure that whatever we do, we do it very cautiously."

"I'll be really honest with you," he said. "I'm glad I don't have to make those decisions."

A Matter of Time

Raul del Toro thought he had a cold.

The 57-year-old National City resident recently lost his job at a hotel in downtown San Diego, he said. By mid-April he was delivering food to people in South County who were too afraid of contracting the virus to visit grocery stores. When he developed a fever and headache, he blamed the heavy rainfall and downed cold medicine at his wife's behest.

As his symptoms grew worse, del Toro visited a clinic in Logan Heights where he tested negative for COVID-19. Days later, he was rushed to a hospital emergency room with a hernia and tested again. It was positive.

Del Toro quarantined himself in his house while his wife looked after him. But as his fever slowly improved, she became ill. On May 3, she tested positive for COVID-19.

"She is small, very tiny. Her body is weaker, so she complains more that she is hurting, that she is more sensitive to everything," he said in Spanish. "She doesn't want to eat. I motivate her to eat more and tell her that her body will have more strength to overcome it. Everything is a matter of time, and your body starts to get over it."

Del Toro won't go back to delivering food—the risk of spreading the virus to others isn't worth taking, he said. For now, he stays home, caring for his wife from a safe distance and disinfecting the house the best he can.

Born in Mexico but now a U.S. citizen, del Toro worries that National City residents are too eager to cross the border into Tijuana, where the virus is circulating quickly, and they aren't taking the risk seriously enough. If the county's stay-at-home restrictions are lifted, he said, even more people will catch it.

"It's too fast because every day there's more cases," del Toro said. "People think this is over, and people are not taking the precautions needed. If people don't wait a bit longer, this is going to get even worse."

National City was the first municipality in the county to require face coverings in public, followed days later by Chula Vista. The leaders of South County cities have called out the county and state for neglecting their residents as cases rise and testing lags.

Chula Vista Mayor Mary Salas told inewsource she attributes her city's growing numbers to its socioeconomic disparities and high volume of essential workers.

"They're working out of necessity, and they're also working because we continue to demand their services," Salas said. Sanitation, healthcare, and restaurant workers are still moving about, she said.

Salas's family has lived in the South Bay for more than 100 years. With a population topping a quarter-million people, more than half of them Hispanic, Chula Vista is reeling from COVID-19.

"Certainly our poorest communities are more severely impacted, and that's been historically the case," said Salas.

The mayor dreads reading the daily tallies of new deaths and infections in her city.

"Is this going to level off? Can we see a drop?" she asked in late April as she reviewed the numbers. "But so far, that's not happening."

When asked this week about the high rate of COVID-19 infections among Hispanic people, Wooten, the county public health officer, said, "I really don't think much should be read into that."

Wooten also said the county is adding more testing sites in vulnerable communities. It opened a new location in Chula Vista last week that doesn't require a doctor's referral.

Even so, the county is far from meeting its goal. As of Friday, San Diego County was reporting results from 3,572 COVID-19 tests. Its target, based on Harvard University estimates, is 5,200 tests a day.

While the county has cited a downward trend in the number of positive COVID-19 tests as justification for reopening, Chula Vista's numbers are still climbing.

On Friday, the city reopened its parks and trails for passive use.

Salas said her community is coming together, with residents doing their best to volunteer and share their resources. A local landscaper donated 200 plants for residents, she said, so when she goes on food donation runs, she drops off a plant.

"The food to nourish their bodies, the plants to remind them that we do live in a beautiful world," she said.

"And we are going to appreciate that world more than ever once we climb out of this."

Inewsource staff member Carla Sánchez contributed to this story

Jill Castellano and Mary Plummer

Why Some COVID-19 Victims Are Dying at Home Without Medical Care

> This story was originally produced and published by inewsource, a nonprofit, nonpartisan newsroom in San Diego committed to exposing wrongdoing and holding powerful people and institutions accountable. As part of their commitment to keeping the San Diego community informed, inewsource has allowed this story to be reprinted and shared here with you. To learn more about their work and how you can support their journalism, visit inewsource.org.

September 3, 2020

A 44-year-old woman was tested for COVID-19 at the Palomar Medical Center in Escondido. She was found unresponsive in bed three days later while waiting for her results.

In Chula Vista, a 54-year-old man who had been sick for two weeks stayed home rather than seek medical care. His roommate found him on the toilet, deceased.

And an El Centro man with kidney disease was denied dialysis twice after developing a fever and coronavirus symptoms. Days later, he fell out of his car and went to the hospital, where he tested positive for the virus. He was sent home and died soon after at UCSD Medical Center.

These stories reflect the growing number of people in the region who are not getting the medical attention they need until it's too late.

Deaths at home have climbed to levels well above what San Diego County has seen in the prior three years, according to an inewsource review of public health data. The percentage of deaths occurring in homes—as opposed to in hospitals or other settings—rose from 34.8% in 2019 to about 38% since January.

Andrew Noymer, an epidemiologist at UC Irvine who studies pandemics, said the findings "highlight a gap" in communication from public officials to residents about the virus and when to seek help.

While there's no way of knowing for sure if a hospital visit will save a life, Noymer said, in some cases, it could.

"People need to understand that if they're very sick, they need to seek medical care," he said.

Interviews with healthcare workers, researchers, and the families of those who have died shed light on why some who are seriously ill are not going to hospitals: a belief that doctors can't or won't help COVID-19 patients, a lack of education and guidance from public health workers, and an ongoing problem with false-negative test results.

Totally Alone

Hector Navarro Lopez, who died from the virus after his wife called 911 from their house, hadn't seen a doctor since 2018.

The 52-year-old San Marcos resident had worked two jobs—in manufacturing and newspaper distribution—to provide for his wife and four children, but it still wasn't enough. He had let his health insurance lapse for six months to save money.

Noemi Arroyo Ramirez, his wife of 26 years, said he had no underlying health conditions and was almost never sick, so he rarely took the time for routine checkups.

On May 18, after developing a mild cough and difficulty tasting food, Navarro Lopez went to a county lab for a COVID-19 test, his wife said, but he wouldn't get the results for four days.

In the meantime, he experienced stomach discomfort and an occasional fever. He sought help from North County Health Services in San

Marcos, a nonprofit clinic that predominantly serves low-income and Hispanic families.

At the clinic, staff were screening patients for coronavirus symptoms and taking their temperatures before allowing anyone to enter the building.

When Arroyo told the healthcare workers that her husband had a fever the day before, she said the employees abruptly packed up their belongings and retreated inside the clinic. Roughly 10 minutes later, a worker returned, telling the family to go home and wait for a call from a doctor.

Areli, the couple's oldest child, said it felt like the staff had no compassion for her dad once they thought he might have the virus.

"People don't know how to handle it," the 24-year-old said. "They enter this paranoia. There's no respect."

She added: "I can't help but think maybe they didn't do enough."

The ailing father received a phone call later that day from the clinic. Arroyo said the doctor didn't ask to see her husband's stomach over video chat and offered no medication or treatments—only instructions to call back once Navarro Lopez's test results came in.

The following day, on May 22, he got the news: positive for COVID-19.

Arroyo called the clinic and left a message, she said, but never heard back.

In a statement, Dr. Marie Russell, the North County Health Services chief medical officer, said its clinics have been "committed to caring for the community throughout the COVID-19 pandemic" and began screening patients for symptoms early on to protect others from the virus.

Russell said if someone tests positive at their designated labs, a doctor will follow up and provide care instructions. But in Navarro Lopez's case, he was tested at a different lab before he ever walked into the San Marcos clinic.

A spokesperson for the clinic added that its doctors strive to do video appointments when they can't see patients in person, but sometimes phone visits are necessary if there are technical difficulties or the patient has "limited video capability."

Arroyo said she was left to care for her husband using her own intuition, television, and Google search results.

She gave him hot tea, isolated him in a bedroom, took his temperature multiple times a day and supplied him with aspirin, vitamin C, and Tylenol.

But Arroyo is no doctor. She didn't know that the coronavirus can cause oxygen levels to drop dangerously low even while someone looks and acts normal.

And she didn't know what to do when her husband's fever rose to 103 degrees. All she saw in online articles was to go to the hospital if your temperature reaches 104.

"It felt like, 'This is your patient. Take care of him. It's your responsibility. If he passes away, it's your fault,'" Arroyo said.

"I felt like that, like I'm alone. Totally alone."

Arroyo said after losing her husband to COVID-19, she lost her trust in healthcare providers, too.

"If I feel like I will die, I will go to the hospital," she said. "Otherwise, I will not go to a hospital or talk to a doctor because they don't help me with something simple [like] stomach problems."

A Devastating Outcome

Reports from the San Diego County medical examiner's office tell the stories of more than a dozen COVID-19 victims since March who died at home or on their way to hospitals.

In five cases, the victims tried to seek medical care in their final hours before death but could not be saved. In another four, they were rushed across the border from Mexico in search of an ambulance. In three, they suffered serious falls—a common side effect of the virus in old age—that resulted in their deaths.

Four other reports say the deceased were found unresponsive at home by family members, roommates, or others.

The medical examiner's office only reviews a small fraction of COVID-19 cases, including sometimes when the cause of death is unclear or when the victim hasn't sought medical care recently. The reports grimly describe how the virus can attack the body at full force without warning, and how quickly it can take a life—especially when medical professionals aren't available to help.

Experts say a reticence to seek medical care can result from misunderstandings about how American hospitals are operating during the pandemic.

This is especially true in border communities. Dr. Eva Tovar Hirashima, the prehospital medical director at the Tijuana Red Cross and an emergency room doctor in Riverside, said people who have previously sought medical care in Mexico may expect a similar experience in the U.S.—that hospitals are too overwhelmed to take care of patients who aren't visibly, seriously ill.

"People who are first generation [Americans] and who have been exposed to the Mexican medical system may believe that in order for them to actually be assessed appropriately and admitted to the hospital, they really need to come at the last minute," Tovar Hirashima said.

"Because if they don't come at the last minute, then they'll be discharged home."

Early on in the pandemic, Tovar Hirashima realized that more Tijuana residents asking for medical help from the Red Cross were dead by the time emergency paramedic teams arrived on the scene.

San Diego physicians noticed something similar on the U.S. side of the border—the number of emergency room patients was shrinking, not growing.

County data shows that early on in the pandemic, roughly 48,000 fewer people visited the region's emergency rooms than during that time in 2019.

Meanwhile, home deaths started to rise. Hundreds more people in San Diego County have died in their homes than would be expected in a normal year, according to a review of county public health data.

By April, hospital executives were appealing to the public through the news media, encouraging people to seek medical attention if they felt unwell.

"Our concern is the patients that do have chest pain or stroke symptoms—if they're waiting to come in, time is literally ticking away," Dr. Ghazala Sharieff, the chief medical officer of Scripps Health, told KUSI News in April. "So if they wait, that could be a devastating outcome."

Dr. Wilma Wooten, the county's public health officer, said officials are educating the public through their healthcare partners, media sources, and other channels to alleviate concerns about the coronavirus. She encouraged residents to reach out to their physicians if they don't feel well.

"Don't be afraid to seek healthcare," Wooten said. "Call your doctor. Much of medical care is being conducted via telemedicine. So in many cases you may not need to go in face-to-face."

But Wooten's statement didn't acknowledge the many San Diegans without a regular primary care physician to call. Navarro Lopez, the San Marcos resident, was one of them.

In county survey results from 2015, about 14% of San Diegans said they did not have a regular place to go when they became sick, and 18% had not visited a doctor in the past year.

Gene Kallenberg, a faculty physician at UC San Diego, said primary care doctors are a key source of support and guidance for COVID-19 patients. Not having one is frequently the root of the problem, he said.

"Potentially the absence of a relationship with a primary care physician led to the patients making these poor judgments that left them home in bed and dying," Kallenberg said.

At UCSD, doctors communicate with their coronavirus patients almost every day until they recover, Kallenberg said.

"It's tragic to me when someone has no one to call," he said.

Playing Catch-Up

If a resident with COVID-19 doesn't have a regular primary care provider, the county tries to fill in the gap.

The county public health office says it has multiple "touchpoints" to communicate with coronavirus-positive residents and provide them with care instructions.

But some people—like Navarro Lopez and his family—get left behind.

The first point of contact occurs when a person tests positive for the virus at a public lab. A county nurse is supposed to reach out to them with instructions for isolating at home, wearing a mask, social distancing, and disinfecting their environment. The nurse is also supposed to explain when it might be necessary to go to the hospital.

Arroyo said her husband was tested at a county-run lab in Escondido, and yet the family never received a call.

The second touchpoint occurs during contact tracing. Public officials say case investigators try to reach everyone who tests positive for COVID-19, so they can track down others who were potentially exposed. Then, a separate group of workers called contact tracers reach out to those who may have been infected.

The process poses another opportunity for the public to speak with experts about what they should do to protect themselves and monitor their health. But Arroyo said she and her husband did not receive calls from investigators or contact tracers.

County Supervisor Nathan Fletcher, who co-chairs the region's COVID-19 taskforce, said he didn't know the details of Navarro Lopez's case, but it's possible the county could have had outdated or incorrect phone numbers for the family.

Rick Greenwood, a member of California's testing taskforce, said case investigators and contact tracers up and down the state are swamped with work. The problem with contact tracing, he said, is the more tests that are conducted, the more the staff becomes overwhelmed.

"If you only do a thousand tests and find a few people positive, the system isn't stressed," Greenwood said. "If you start doing 200,000 and 300,000 a day and end up with thousands of positives, you need to have a system in place to know what to do with them."

"The state's playing catch-up," he added, "trying to hire people at the same time that hundreds of positive tests are coming in."

In San Diego County, contact tracing efforts slowed in late July. At the time, the county's goal was for 70% of investigations to begin within 24 hours, but only 11% did.

Fletcher said the county has hired additional staff and now has a big enough team to reach everyone who has tested positive and the people they could have infected.

As of late August, 97% of investigations are opened within one day, and more than 40,000 investigations have been performed, public health data shows.

"The aim and intention is to contact all," the supervisor said. "And that's how we're structured. That's how we're staffed. That's how we're set up. And that's how we're operating."

Of the people local investigators reach out to, 90% have provided information to the contact tracing team. That leaves 10%—or 3,472 people—who could not be reached or would not answer questions as of mid-August, including Navarro Lopez's family.

With no experts to turn to for advice, Navarro Lopez's wife didn't seek medical attention for him until she knew it was an emergency.

On the morning of May 27, her husband told her something was wrong with his legs.

"I feel bad. I feel bad," Navarro Lopez repeated.

Arroyo called 911, but by the time an ambulance arrived her husband insisted he was better and didn't want to go to the hospital.

She begged.

Arroyo told her husband this might be their one chance to finally hear from a healthcare worker about his illness and how she should be taking care of him.

Navarro Lopez obliged his wife's pleas, walking to the stretcher. He had two heart attacks before he made it to Palomar hospital.

The day he died, Navarro Lopez left behind a son finishing ninth grade, a daughter graduating high school in two weeks, a son in college with dreams of working in the Sheriff's Department and a 24-year-old daughter less than two months away from getting married.

The family's cozy San Marcos home is copiously decorated with sports trophies, framed photos, school awards, woodworking projects, and religious icons. Gathered together there in late July, Navarro Lopez's four children and their mom held each other close, crying and laughing as they remembered their beloved patriarch.

"We're gonna use my father as something that's going to propel us forward and for us to succeed," said Hector, 22.

Miranda, 17, called her dad a "man above all men" with a pure heart. Axel, 15, said nobody ever had anything bad to say about his father.

Areli, 24, described her father as a quiet man who protected and guided the family.

"I knew that with him and my mom around as our parents, everything was going to be okay and everything was going to be possible," she said.

The loss taught her that sometimes the only way to survive is to be resourceful, Areli said.

"If somebody doesn't want to help you, find a way to help yourself."

Testing the System

Alfonso Ye Jr., a 25-year-old part-time pharmacy technician, tried to get help when he started feeling sick.

On March 17, he went to Scripps Memorial Hospital in San Diego and tested negative for the virus, according to coroner's records. The hospital diagnosed him with a respiratory infection and gave him no medication, the records say.

Not long after his discharge, the El Cajon resident headed to Riverside County to stay at his mom's house in La Quinta until he felt better.

Eight days later, when he had trouble breathing, his mother wanted him to go to the hospital, according to the coroner's records, but Ye repeatedly said his COVID-19 test was negative and did not go.

Ye's mom called 911. The paramedics couldn't save him.

A posthumous test confirmed the pharmacy student was positive for the coronavirus. The coroner's records said he died from respiratory distress caused by COVID-19, making him one of the first documented San Diego County residents to die from the virus.

Tools to detect the coronavirus aren't advanced enough to decipher whether someone like Ye developed the virus after testing negative or if his first test result was inaccurate.

As the number of COVID-19 tests conducted continues to rise, so do the number of false-negative results, which can discourage someone from seeking potentially life-saving medical care.

A June paper from the Mayo Clinic estimated there could be more than 20,000 people in California who received false-negative results. The scientists warned that if healthcare providers aren't careful in interpreting test results and advising patients, it could cause someone to develop a dangerous confidence that they are virus-free.

Research from Johns Hopkins found that COVID-19 tests working at their best still lead to false negatives about 20% of the time, meaning at least 1 in 5 people with the virus receive negative test results.

The Food and Drug Administration cautions healthcare providers that false-negative tests can lead to a delayed diagnosis and improper treatment. Plus, they can result in patients failing to monitor their symptoms closely.

In a June fact sheet, the federal agency advised that when a patient tests negative, medical workers should consider the likelihood that the person was exposed to the virus when deciding how reliable the test results are.

In Ye's case, he had a colleague who had recently tested positive for the virus and was on a ventilator, according to what his mother told the coroner's office.

A spokesperson for Scripps Health declined an interview request and did not comment specifically on Ye or his test results. He said the hospital system has no way of knowing how often negative COVID-19 tests are tied to individuals who later test positive.

Ye's death was a loss upon loss for his family. His father, of the same name, died about two years ago.

Stephanie Silva, Ye Jr.'s cousin, said Ye was very ambitious and his life was going well. He loved his job and was planning to graduate from the pharmacy program at Pima Medical Institute in Chula Vista in April. He was living in El Cajon with a roommate, his first time venturing away from home in a big way.

Ye loved San Diego's live-music scene and Disneyland, his cousin said. He was someone people always looked forward to seeing and someone who'd go out of his way to visit friends and family.

"He was always the go-to person for anyone that wanted to just talk," Silva said. "He was the person that you wanted to talk to if you were feeling sad."

Ye was well liked and high achieving. He'd applied for and earned his pharmacy technician license while still in school, a step that showed his initiative, said Benjamin Montoya, one of his professors.

"He was young. He was full of life," Montoya said. "He had so much in front of him. It really hit me hard."

It's been almost six months since Silva lost her cousin. She said his death and the other lives lost to the pandemic feel like they could have been avoided if more safety precautions had been in place.

"It's very sad how many people see these numbers but don't really see the people behind them," she said.

Inewsource intern Sofía Mejías-Pascoe and reporter Camille von Kaenel contributed to this story

Jill Castellano
Remembering the Human Toll of COVID-19 in San Diego County

> *This story was originally produced and published by inewsource, a nonprofit, nonpartisan newsroom in San Diego committed to exposing wrongdoing and holding powerful people and institutions accountable. As part of their commitment to keeping the San Diego community informed, inewsource has allowed this story to be reprinted and shared here with you. To learn more about their work and how you can support their journalism, visit inewsource.org.*

December 23, 2020

We all know this hasn't been an easy year.

When San Diego County first imposed stay-at-home orders in March, officials said they hoped the region would return to some semblance of normalcy within a few weeks. Nine months later, now on our second lockdown order, COVID-19 cases and deaths are skyrocketing.

Currently, 0% of Southern California's ICU beds are available as more people are hospitalized with the virus. Already, more than 1,200 county residents have died from COVID-19.

Underneath the hospitalization rates and death statistics are people who have suffered, sacrificed, lost lives, and lost loved ones. At inewsource, we've spent the past nine months bringing you the stories that show the human toll COVID-19 has taken on our communities.

We recently caught up with some of the families who lost relatives and friends this year—families that generously opened their homes and their hearts to our reporters and told us their stories. In a holiday season like no other in recent memory, they told us they are still looking for ways to cope and celebrate the people they lost to the coronavirus.

"We've been literally torn apart from each other and just waiting, waiting, waiting for a time when we can be together," said Vicki Sutherland, who lost her father, Joe Villegas, and aunt, Mona Weiss, to COVID-19.

Sutherland, who spoke with us for a story on challenges with COVID-19 treatment and testing in July, hasn't seen her extended family since the deaths occurred. She's holding onto her father's ashes and hopes to plan a memorial service sometime in 2021.

"That's almost the harder part, not being able to grieve and celebrate life," she said.

As a part of our July story, five families shared what happened leading up to their relatives' deaths and how those deaths may have been avoidable. We followed up with another project in September, exploring the fears and other obstacles that prevented COVID-19 victims from seeking potentially life-saving medical care.

After that, we reported on the other deaths caused by the pandemic—the people who never contracted COVID-19 but are considered "indirect" victims of the virus: the mother of a 22-year-old who suffered a drug overdose, the brother of a heart attack victim, and the daughter of a polio survivor. Each one told us how the pandemic changed their loved ones' lives, mental states, and workout routines, ultimately leading to their deaths.

One thing connects all the families we spoke with for our pandemic stories this year: They are still grappling with the unexpected losses of cherished family members.

For Sutherland, one thing that has helped her stay positive was building an altar for her father on the Day of the Dead. It helped her connect with her Hispanic and Mexican heritage, she said, and the family found it very therapeutic.

But Thanksgiving was more challenging. Usually, about 20 of her relatives would get together to laugh, eat, and drink, but this year she stayed home with her husband and daughter.

One of the lessons she told us she's learned through all this is "how important family is to me."

"I cannot wait to get a hold of these people and give them a hug and a kiss," Sutherland said.

Our reporting this year has explored just how difficult isolation caused by the pandemic has been. Assisted living facilities and nursing homes have banned visitors during most of the pandemic to keep residents safe. But experts say family members are the best advocates for the residents to ensure they're receiving proper care, and things can go seriously wrong when they're not present.

Even with visitor bans, the virus has crippled San Diego County's long-term care facilities. More than 1,600 healthcare workers and 1,900 patients have contracted COVID-19 at the county's nursing homes.

At one assisted living home in Chula Vista, five of six residents tested positive for the virus and three died in the first three months of the pandemic.

Rebecca Niebla's grandmother died of COVID-19 at Windsor Gardens, a National City nursing home. We spoke with her in July about how staffing shortages left these facilities unprepared to tackle the pandemic.

She couldn't visit her grandmother, Esther Hernandez, in the weeks leading up to her death. At the time, Niebla said the nursing home didn't take the right precautions and believed the facility could have prevented her grandmother from catching the virus.

Now, she's trying to put those thoughts behind her.

"It wasn't healthy for us to keep digging and finding out the details," she said. "It was better for us to let go and start healing."

Niebla and her 6-year-old son moved in with her mother to support each other during the pandemic. Together, they help each other remember all the wonderful things about Esther.

"She had a full life," her granddaughter said. "She was very healthy. She loved her family. So we just have to move on with our lives and continue with her legacy."

Jennifer Bowman

Even With Vaccines, San Diego's Vulnerable Communities Still Report High COVID-19 Rates

> *This story was originally produced and published by inewsource, a nonprofit, nonpartisan newsroom in San Diego committed to exposing wrongdoing and holding powerful people and institutions accountable. As part of their commitment to keeping the San Diego community informed, inewsource has allowed this story to be reprinted and shared here with you. To learn more about their work and how you can support their journalism, visit inewsource.org.*

December 15, 2021

Ana Melgoza remembers vividly the pandemic's early days in South County.

"When you look at who died because of this and also in terms of the impact at ER rooms and ICU rooms—I mean, we were seeing waits of, like, three days to get into a hospital," said Melgoza, vice president of external affairs at San Ysidro Health. "We were very much in high turmoil."

The South Bay quickly became the hardest-hit part of San Diego County as COVID-19 shut down schools and businesses almost two years ago. Now, it boasts the highest vaccination rates in the region and has served as a model for administering doses to vulnerable populations.

But that hasn't quelled transmission. As the vast majority of the county continues to grapple with high or substantial COVID-19 numbers, the most vulnerable neighborhoods—including those in the South Bay—are still being disproportionately impacted.

Nearly all eligible residents in San Ysidro's 92173 ZIP code have received at least one COVID-19 vaccine dose. But the area is still reporting daily an average of more than 30 cases per 100,000 residents, the highest rate in the county.

Other areas that were deemed vulnerable by state officials during the pandemic have the county's second-highest rates: A combination of six ZIP codes comprising the backcountry communities of Jacumba, Campo and Boulevard, along with the 92113 ZIP code that includes Lincoln Park, Logan Heights, and Barrio Logan, are reporting about 23 cases per 100,000 residents a day.

Those who have worked in the county's early hotspots say the cases show which residents remain at highest risk: essential workers, public transit users, undocumented residents, and members of multigenerational households.

Most often, they're people of color, said Elisa Sobo, professor and chair of anthropology at San Diego State University.

"And in San Diego, of course that means Hispanic people," she said. "The chance for exposure, whether you're vaccinated or not, it's much, much higher than for someone who's able to telecommute."

While vaccinations clearly play a role in keeping people out of the hospital and avoiding severe infection, even in highly vaccinated ZIP codes there are people at risk: immunocompromised residents, children who until recently didn't have access to vaccinations, and those who haven't received any of the shots.

"I worry about all of those people," said Corinne McDaniels-Davidson, director of SDSU's Institute for Public Health. "On top of that, I also worry because when you have high transmission, that's when the variants can emerge."

As health officials across the U.S. continue to monitor the omicron variant—with the first case in San Diego confirmed last week—experts say the answers may lie in successful efforts first started in South County: Community partnerships helped boost vaccination rates there and could be exported to parts of the backcountry where numbers are lagging even amid high transmission.

But vaccinations still will need to be coupled with other public health interventions, McDaniels-Davidson said, like well-ventilated buildings and masks. Citing a 47% increase in infection rates since Thanksgiving, the state announced that residents—even those fully vaccinated—must again wear masks in all indoor public settings. The mandate is in place until January. 15.

"Vaccines are critical," McDaniels-Davidson said. "They are so critical, and they are so important at stopping the disease—meaning the terrible sickness that can happen after someone is infected—but they can't be our only strategy to stopping infection."

Where Transmission Is High

As COVID-19 vaccines became more widely available, the state in March rolled out a new equity plan to provide extra doses in some of the most vulnerable communities. At the time, they had suffered 40% of cases and deaths during the pandemic.

Officials cited their status as having among the poorest access in the state to healthy conditions: They fell in the bottom 25% of the state's Healthy Places Index, which considers factors such as employment, educational level, air quality and household crowding, among others.

A dozen ZIP codes were identified in San Diego, spanning from the county's rural neighborhoods like Warner Springs and Dulzura to densely populated areas such as City Heights and San Ysidro.

But as of December 8, seven of the 12 ZIP codes were experiencing high transmission, and three others were faring slightly better with substantial transmission. (Rates for the remaining two ZIP codes were censored by the county due to their small case numbers.)

Just six areas in San Diego were reporting moderate transmission: Coronado; Hillcrest; 92111 in Kearny Mesa, Clairemont, and Linda Vista; La Jolla's 92037, Carlsbad's 92011; and two ZIP codes that include Bonsall and Vista. There is no part of the county that is reporting what would qualify as low transmission.

McDaniels-Davidson said even in areas with the highest vaccination rates, many still "don't actually have a lot of choice in those other things that they're doing."

"They don't have a choice in where they work or how safe that workplace is, or how much of the public they come into contact with," she said. "So when you're talking about lower wage workers, they don't have a lot of protections against transmission."

As experts and advocates had feared, the South Bay and its large share of Latino residents suffered some of the worst numbers as high transmission coupled with poverty and disparities in preexisting health conditions. Several months into the pandemic, a CalMatters report found Latino children were testing positive at higher rates than other groups of kids, with experts citing more crowded living conditions and close contact with essential workers.

The pandemic amplified an economic crisis that many South Bay families were already experiencing, San Ysidro Health's Melgoza said. San Ysidro is one of the region's poorest neighborhoods, with a median household income 40% less than that of San Diego citywide.

"We have a lot of families that are barely making it, and there's a lot of ingenious ways to get ahead," Melgoza said. "A lot of it can be a very, health-wise, unstable setting."

All of San Ysidro and much of Chula Vista remain under high transmission, meaning the average daily case rate equals or exceeds 14.3 cases per 100,000 people and that more than 10% of COVID-19 tests are coming back positive.

High transmission also is being reported in the county's backcountry, where most ZIP codes are reporting that fewer than half of eligible residents have been vaccinated. That's despite clear data showing vaccines are crucial: Since March, nearly 83% of the county's COVID-19 deaths have been among people who weren't fully vaccinated.

McDaniels-Davidson said communities with lower vaccination rates are more likely to suffer from "high, severe disease." And unlike South County, other parts of the region may not have a strong system of trusted organizations for engagement and vaccine outreach.

"Those are the places that we really do need to do more work, to have conversations with people about getting vaccinated, to try to kind of stem the tide," she said.

Lessons Learned

Today, health care providers in the county are no longer struggling with limited protective equipment or testing access. Hospitalizations are drastically down from a year ago. Three-fourths of eligible residents are fully vaccinated against COVID-19, outpacing the statewide rate. Hispanics and Latinos, disproportionately impacted by the pandemic, are reporting a nearly 73% vaccination rate in the county.

"What we have learned from COVID is that thinking outside the box, breaking down barriers and creating interventions that really work for communities that are on the front lines can really make a difference," said county Supervisor Nora Vargas, who represents the southern region and took office in January.

South County became a starting point for several successful initiatives during the pandemic: One of the first local supersites for vaccinations was set up inside a former Sears at the Chula Vista Center mall. Promotoras, or community health workers who are well-trusted in Latino communities, worked closely with local supermarkets to make vaccines available without appointments.

Experts credit the well-established relationships that community organizations had with residents, some of them wary of interacting with government officials or lacking prior access to health care. An October report by CommuniVax, a national coalition of educators and advocates that includes SDSU's Sobo and McDaniels-Davidson, recommended other regions with a high proportion of Hispanic and Latino residents follow South County's successes.

Sobo, the SDSU professor, acknowledged the differences among communities but said some of the strategies that worked in South County can be borrowed for other parts of San Diego, too.

"If you're talking about a population that's not Hispanic, you can still have the promotora model," she said. "You just wouldn't call it that. It's just a matter of having people who are insiders be there to provide information, to provide assistance and help get questions answered."

McDaniels-Davidson admits that work may be harder in other parts of the county.

"Especially in rural parts of the county," she said. "You have to figure out who's trusted and why they're trusted. And then you have to work through them."

Roxana Popescu, Mary Plummer, and Jill Castellano

Coronavirus Deaths: San Diego Families Grapple With Mistakes, Slow Testing, and Poor Care

> *This story was originally produced and published by inewsource, a nonprofit, nonpartisan newsroom in San Diego committed to exposing wrongdoing and holding powerful people and institutions accountable. As part of their commitment to keeping the San Diego community informed, inewsource has allowed this story to be reprinted and shared here with you. To learn more about their work and how you can support their journalism, visit inewsource.org.*

July 15, 2020

To their families, they were the teacher with sparkling eyes and a love for bocce ball. The keen student of history who had survived a U.S. internment camp for Japanese Americans. The dad to a 9-year-old. The wife of 59 years.

They are now, also, absences and enigmas.

In San Diego County, more than 400 lives have been lost to the new coronavirus since the pandemic struck the region in March, and the crisis is far from over. As San Diegans venture out into public spaces and some resume normal activities, infections are on the rise and people keep dying.

As of Monday, about 44% of those who died in San Diego County were Hispanic or Latino, inewsource found. A third who died were from South County, 56% were male, and 87% were over 60 years old. A striking 95% of those who died had underlying health conditions.

In interviews with inewsource, families of the deceased brought up multiple issues that led to the worst outcome for these patients: a veteran didn't receive a potentially lifesaving plasma therapy on time because the supply was tainted; a woman likely caught the virus from home healthcare workers who tended to her ailing husband; one man was denied testing, despite being sick enough that he died soon after; another contracted the virus while living at a memory care facility; and a merchant mariner was asked to work on a Navy ship without adequate precautions.

Here are their stories. There are hundreds of others—healthcare workers, the disease's youngest victims, the people experiencing homelessness, those who contracted the virus in San Diego and died in Mexico, the people who were never tested or counted—and the list keeps growing. So does the list of unanswered questions.

Death 99: Tainted Plasma

After testing positive for COVID-19, 43-year-old veteran Robert Mendoza drove himself to Tri-City Medical Center in Oceanside, suffering from low oxygen levels. The doctors almost didn't admit him because his symptoms didn't seem severe, Mendoza's parents said—he could still talk and walk fine on his own. But they eventually found him a bed.

He was admitted to the hospital on a Monday in April. About two days later, he was placed in the ICU.

He died five days after that.

"I really—from Monday to Wednesday, I ask myself what could have happened," said his mother, Yolanda Mendoza.

Her son was known as a fighter and a survivor. He left home at 17 to fulfill his dream of joining the Marines, eventually traveling to Iraq and Afghanistan for battle. After a parachuting accident caused a broken femur and pelvis, doctors inserted a titanium rod into his leg. He rejoined the military after mastering a grueling series of physical tests.

Mendoza's father, who is also named Robert, said he couldn't believe "that somebody could go through three wars and survive and come home, and then something you can't even see can take them down."

One thing the veteran's parents hoped would improve his condition came too late: Mendoza had been approved for a plasma therapy, his parents said, but when the plasma arrived at the hospital it was "tainted" and couldn't be used. Mendoza's mother said she was given the news by the hospital's charge nurse, but nobody explained to her how the shipment became contaminated.

The next order of plasma wasn't delivered for another day or two, and by then the father of a 9-year-old boy was on dialysis for kidney failure. He died the next morning, on April 20.

"It just makes me wonder if he had received the plasma when he went into the ICU on Wednesday, or maybe if he had received it on Thursday or Friday, maybe the outcome would have been different," Yolanda Mendoza said.

Tri-City Medical Center confirmed in a statement that the hospital is partnering with the Mayo Clinic to offer convalescent plasma therapy, an experimental treatment in which people who have recovered from the coronavirus donate their blood plasma to those who are still sick. The hope is that the antibodies could help severely ill patients like Mendoza fight off the infection.

Aaron Byzak, chief external affairs officer for Tri-City Medical Center, said the hospital can't comment on what happened in Mendoza's case because of health privacy concerns. But he said, "Plasma containing certain antibodies may not be used due to potential harmful effects."

Though the benefits of plasma therapy haven't been proven, preliminary research shows some patients have reported positive responses.

As a part of his treatment, Mendoza did receive hydroxychloroquine, a malaria drug President Donald Trump has touted to fight the coronavirus. The Food and Drug Administration briefly authorized the use of the drug for COVID-19 patients but revoked that authorization in June because of emerging evidence that it does not help people who have the virus—and it may even harm them.

As his health worsened, Mendoza's parents kept calling the hospital to speak with their son. But the busy healthcare workers on the other end were only able to put him on the phone one time, for a video call minutes before his death.

He couldn't speak, and his parents don't know if he could hear them saying they loved him.

At Mendoza's small funeral in Houston, Marines served as pallbearers. His parents have received phone calls from veterans across the globe who served alongside their son, telling them how much they loved him.

"My son had a lot of friends," Robert Mendoza said. "But I just didn't realize how many he had."

Death 248: "Little Cracks"

Kent Yamada had built what he thought was a fortress around his elderly parents, with meticulous practices around distancing, disinfection, and isolation.

Despite the family's efforts, Kent Yamada said "little cracks" appeared. At first, they were invisible. Then they couldn't be unseen.

He believes his mother, Elizabeth Kikuchi-Yamada, contracted the virus from any of the dozen or so healthcare workers who came and left their La Jolla home in March and April to help his father, Joseph Yamada, who had severe dementia.

One man came to talk about getting a hospital-grade bed for Joseph. Two other workers followed up, taking measurements, and a different team delivered it. Another healthcare worker brought oxygen to the house. EMTs entered at one point, and medical educators visited another time to talk with Elizabeth about her husband's condition.

Some of these people wore masks. Some did not.

Each visitor, and each lapse, added to the risk of infection for Elizabeth and Joseph. Both were 90.

Yamada said he would ask the healthcare workers to put on masks. EMTs wore gloves and other protective gear, but the others did not.

His mother, who he described as "fit as a horse," didn't understand how easily the virus could spread—she called it "the COVID" and thought it was a type of flu. But Yamada believes the home health workers should have known better and taken more precautions.

"When you're thinking that you're working with healthcare people, you really do believe that they're professionals and they wouldn't do anything to endanger or take a risk," Yamada said. "But the truth is that they aren't as serious as you think they are."

California passed a law in 2016 requiring home care aides to pass background checks and enter an online registry. The state's Home Care Services Bureau also regulates the care provided by these aides, responds to complaints, and conducts unannounced inspections.

In response to the pandemic, the bureau recommended in April that home care aides wear face coverings, not work if they are sick, disinfect objects in the home they're working in, and avoid physical contact with patients when possible. If a client has a suspected or confirmed case of COVID-19, aides are supposed to wear medical-grade masks and other protective gear.

But the bureau has also loosened its rules around some inspections and investigations: Rather than conducting them in person, they can occur remotely. A similar change around on-site inspections at nursing homes has outraged advocates, who claim virtual visits aren't enough to make sure the vulnerable and elderly are protected from the virus.

Plus, unlike the staff in nursing homes, home care aides don't have to follow strict testing requirements for COVID-19, increasing the likelihood that asymptomatic workers could carry the virus undetected into their clients' homes.

Khai Nguyen, the clinical services chief for geriatrics at UC San Diego Health, said healthcare workers need better access to coronavirus testing to protect their patients.

"I think 'problem' is an understatement when it comes to testing healthcare workers in general. We need more testing," Nguyen said. "There's no doubt about it."

Elizabeth and Joseph, who was a noted landscape architect, had roughly a dozen contacts in the course of about a month.

Rebecca Fielding-Miller, an assistant professor of infectious disease and global public health at UCSD, said each of those people likely had many other high-risk interactions as part of their jobs. Then they went home and possibly exposed their own relatives and household members.

"Of course [the home health worker] needs to be masking and being careful, but that's a lot of risk for one person to be taking on for $24,000 a year," she said, referring to the average yearly wages for home health aides in 2018. These workers, she added, tend to be from populations that are more affected by the coronavirus, such as immigrants. "There's kind of a compounding of risk," Fielding-Miller said.

Workers need to be trained but also equipped to do their jobs safely by their employers, Fielding-Miller said.

"How many masks is this person being issued a day?" she asked. "Are they being given hand sanitizer that they can take to different sites? Are they being expected to bring their own?"

Kikuchi-Yamada died at Scripps Green Hospital in La Jolla on May 20.

In her 90 years, she had survived an internment camp for Japanese Americans, graduated from UC Berkeley, raised three children, taught English at San Diego High School, led a fulfilling life, and still she wanted to live "just a bit longer" to say goodbye to her friends and family, her son said.

But she was not interested in a life without her husband, who had died in early May from dementia, her son said. The couple had met when they were 11. In the days before Joseph Yamada's death, his wife had snuggled next to him, dozing, and barely eating. The kids thought she was grieving, but she was already sick.

Her death certificate lists three causes: respiratory failure, pneumonia, and COVID-19. When Kent Yamada talks with people about what happened, he tells them his mother died of a broken heart.

Deaths 85 and 297: Testing Delays

The first in the family to die from the virus was Mona Weiss.

The 88-year-old, a great cook known for her albondigas soup and homemade pinto beans, developed a bad cough and was losing her appetite in mid-March. So her son, Michael Weiss, 54, took her to her doctor at a Scripps Health medical building in Chula Vista.

He listened to her lungs and told the mother and son it was bronchitis. The prescription: medication to treat it and self-care at home. Although San Diego County already had several dozen cases of the coronavirus, no X-ray and no COVID-19 test was ordered, Michael said.

The second family member to die, a month and a half after Mona, was Michael's 90-year-old uncle—the husband of Mona's sister. Though Joe Villegas and Mona had not had contact with one another and caught the virus through different channels, a common thread connects their deaths: Both had trouble getting tested for COVID-19.

In the end, COVID-19 infected at least seven members of the Weiss and Villegas families. The virus—combined with inadequate access to testing and other health conditions—cost them two lives.

After Mona was sent home to her house in Chula Vista with a cough, the virus took root, undetected.

By early April, her son, who had taken her to the doctor, also contracted the virus along with her granddaughter's husband, who lived with her.

Michael Weiss said he was initially denied testing when he asked his doctor for it. He ended up spending 21 days at the Sharp Chula Vista hospital, 10 on a ventilator, and sacrificing 28 pounds of muscle mass as he fought the virus. When he was strong enough to hear bad news, he learned his mother had died—and she had died alone—of COVID-19.

For Michael and Mona, testing came too late. Both were eventually tested by the hospitals they went to, and both received their results on April 11, long after their symptoms had started and long after their doctors had first been notified of their health worries.

Nguyen, the geriatrics specialist at UCSD, said testing rates are inadequate, including for older patients who might not appear to be sick with the coronavirus though they are infected.

"We should have low thresholds in checking for COVID-19 in our senior patients," Nguyen said. "Because aging in and of itself is a high-risk factor. The [Centers for Disease Control and Prevention] says that eight out of 10 people who have died from coronavirus have been above the age of 65. That to me is most concerning."

In a statement, a spokesperson for Scripps, the healthcare system where Mona received her care, said patients with symptoms of bronchitis and other lung infection-related diseases are "likely" tested for COVID-19 and that the decision is made by the healthcare provider.

A lifelong resident of South County, Mona first lived in San Ysidro and later moved to Chula Vista, where she was part of one of the first graduating classes of Chula Vista High School and went on to raise a family with her husband, Lee. She and Lee had a bike business for a time, and she ran her own jewelry business. Every year on Mother's Day she gave Michael a gift to celebrate him making her a mother.

"She was very ferocious in the way she loved you," Michael said.

Amidst the grief of losing Mona, the family's problems kept coming—this time when Michael's uncle was denied testing after leaving a hospital stay in mid-May and days later died. Joe Villegas's death certificate lists COVID-19 as the primary cause.

He was taken by ambulance to Sharp Memorial Hospital in San Diego in May, following a fall. Next, he was transferred to the Kaiser Permanente hospital in Kearny Mesa. Before Kaiser discharged him, his wife asked that he be tested for COVID-19.

The couple's daughter said her mom was told there weren't enough tests.

So Villegas went home and had close contact with 10 family members over the Memorial Day weekend.

Because of his wife's fears that he had the virus, Villegas got tested on May 26 at a drive-up CVS testing site. But that same day, his condition worsened—he was having symptoms of a potential brain bleed, his daughter said—and he went back to the Kaiser hospital. He stayed one night and was discharged even though test results had come back and showed he was positive.

"My mom literally asked, 'What am I supposed to do? How do I fix this?'" said Vicki Villegas Sutherland, the couple's daughter. "And there was no answer forthcoming."

By June 2, her father was dead.

Joe, a grocery store manager whose careful financial planning allowed him to retire early and travel widely, died in his bedroom. His family peered through an open window, the granddaughters and extended family crying and laughing and talking with him on his last days. Inside the room were his caretaker, his wife, and his daughter Vicki, who held his hands as he took his final breaths. The three of them tried to recreate a hospital-like setting, wearing PPE and masks. Caring for him required extremely close contact.

Both the caretaker and his wife contracted COVID-19.

Sutherland, a home health nurse, is thankful her dad was able to spend his last days at home but believes his death could have been avoided. The lack of testing caused her family much heartache, she said.

"The last two weeks of his life were just fraught," she said. "I keep thinking, does it really have to be like that?"

In a statement, Kaiser acknowledged it may send some COVID-19 positive patients home if they have mild symptoms, to recover "in isolation from others with regular monitoring by clinicians via phone or other means."

In a follow-up email, a spokesperson said Villegas was tested for COVID-19 during his stay at Sharp and transferred to Kaiser with presumed negative results. During his second hospital stay, Kaiser did test him for COVID-19, she said. She added that Villegas was discharged with instructions and a COVID-19 supply kit.

In initial prepared statements to inewsource given after his family granted permission allowing staff to talk, Kaiser incorrectly stated Villegas's date of death and the Kaiser location where he was twice hospitalized. A spokesperson later acknowledged the mistake after an inquiry from inewsource.

Sharp spokesperson John Cihomsky did not comment on specifics of Villegas's stay but said safety precautions were in place when he was hospitalized for his fall and that exposure to COVID-19 "for patients in that situation would be highly unlikely."

Over email, he added: "Our practice now, and at that time, is to test any patient admitted to our hospital, whether they are symptomatic or asymptomatic."

Death 97: "They Were All Just Blindsided"

Lynn Charles Naibert had a suggestion for his daughter as she helped him settle into a San Diego assisted living and memory care home in January. How about she check in, too?

His worsening dementia meant he was up at night and at risk for wandering, his daughter, Pamela Reeb, 64, said. Stellar Care, a facility near El Cerrito where staff are described "like family" in one testimonial on its website, seemed like a way to keep him safe and improve the quality of his life.

A few months after moving, Naibert, 83, died of COVID-19 on April 20. Since the start of the pandemic, more than 40% of deaths nationwide have been residents of nursing homes and other long-term care facilities.

"The hardest thing for me to do was to take my father and put him into Stellar in January," said his daughter Beverly Naibert, 62, who had cared for him in his home before he moved into Stellar Care, helped by a home health worker. "And then three months later, he's dead. How does that make me feel? I feel horrible. I should have just kept him home."

Lynn Naibert's children said the facility's management didn't let them know he was sick or dying until it was too late, didn't test him for the virus, didn't address his acute health issues before deciding he needed hospice care, and has not answered their questions since his death.

On Monday, Beverly Naibert received some documents from Stellar Care, after requesting all of his files and information about the facility's coronavirus infection and death count. The materials she received, she said, included no temperature readings from early March through April 3, and had no information about several incidents the family had been told about over the phone, including falls in his bedroom and in the hallway.

Reeb, who lives in Montana, said she got a series of phone calls in late March and early April saying her father fell a few times over a few days. And then suddenly, she was told they recommended he be put into hospice.

"And when she said 'hospice,' all the red lights started coming on. And I was like, I didn't quite understand why she would say that," Reeb said.

Lynn Naibert, a former teacher, and perpetual quipster who had raised a family with his wife, Penelope, on a sleepy Bay Park cul-de-sac, tested positive for the coronavirus at the UC San Diego hospital in La Jolla in early April and was admitted. He was allowed to see his son, Paul Naibert, who could offer little tenderness because of social distancing, but he took off his glove to hold his father's hand before he died.

State records show 13 residents at Stellar Care have contracted the virus. Linda Cho, the facility's executive director, declined to comment about the Naiberts's concerns.

"Due to rules and regulations for our residents and families, it is not appropriate for us to respond at this time," she wrote in an email.

Reeb thinks the facility's management meant well but became overwhelmed.

"If you take one care facility and you multiply that by the thousands that are in California, I mean, they were all just blindsided by this thing," she said.

Nguyen, the UCSD geriatrician, said the virus can manifest more stealthily in elderly patients, without a textbook presentation, running its course until the person ends up falling, becoming weak or dehydrated.

"It doesn't come with the usual signs that we think of—shortness of breath, cough, fever, [as] in others that have, essentially stronger immune systems. The whole idea is that we need to be more diligent in making sure we're closely following up with these older patients," he said.

Nguyen added that loved ones and caregivers keeping a close watch on people with Alzheimer's and other neurocognitive disorders can help detect illness. That wasn't possible for Naibert once the facility paused visits to mitigate the spread of the virus.

His daughter Beverly has wondered: Why was she, who was living alone and had been her father's caretaker for years, deemed a greater risk to his health than the staff at Stellar Care?

In their final conversation, Lynn Naibert told Beverly he missed her.

"He wanted to come home," she said. "We couldn't bring him home."

A Death That Wasn't Counted

An unknown number of deaths of local residents with COVID-19 are not captured in the county's official data.

Joseph Bondoc is one of them. He isn't listed in the county data, even though he raised his family in National City and owned their home there for seven years before dying on May 21 while away at work in Massachusetts.

The county says it includes San Diego residents who die out of state in its coronavirus reports. A county spokesperson said because Bondoc died away from home there could be a lag in reporting from that state.

But Bondoc was counted by the military. He was among 24 of 47 crew members from a U.S Navy Military Sealift Command ship who tested positive, and the only one who died from the coronavirus. His death was the first of a civilian merchant mariner. The outbreak on the USNS Leroy Grumman—which was in dry dock in Boston and undergoing regularly scheduled maintenance—was among several the military struggled to contain as the pandemic took hold this spring.

Bondoc, who had retired from the Navy, left for Boston on March 24 in good health, aside from high blood pressure and cholesterol issues he'd been managing. He was in the middle of a vacation, sheltering in place at home in National City with his wife and three children.

When he left, his wife, Witchelda Bondoc, wondered why the Military Sealift Command was sending crews to Boston—then a hotspot for the virus—and whether he'd be safe. But her husband took precautions. He saw his doctor before he left, getting refills on his prescriptions and lab work done. He called his wife from aboard the plane as he departed, telling her everyone was wearing masks and social distancing.

About a month into his work assignment, he started feeling sick and developed a fever, so he got tested at a VA hospital. It was, as Witchelda had feared, positive. He was told to self-quarantine and placed under the care of the VA at the hotel where he and other crew members were staying.

A few days later, he left the hotel in an ambulance and was taken to Carney Hospital, a for-profit medical center in Boston that was partially converted to a coronavirus treatment facility.

About 2,500 miles away, Witchelda stayed optimistic. She ordered her husband vitamins and asked her family in the Philippines to prepare special herbs to help him gain his strength when he got home. The couple talked frequently on FaceTime. Each day she handwrote notes on her husband's health in her calendar: May 1, ICU; May 2, lungs weak; May 3, weaker.

They had a video call on May 4, and then Joseph was sedated and put on a ventilator. They wouldn't speak again. Bondoc was buried at Miramar National Cemetery. A ceremony with military honors took place on June 30. It would have been his 55th birthday.

The Military Sealift Command declined inewsource's interview request. In a statement, a spokesperson said the organization's tactics to fight the virus evolved as they learned more, but repair work had to continue.

"While MSC executed its responsibility to protect the health of the MSC crews, there remained a continuing responsibility to maintain MSC ships to perform their national security missions," the statement said.

It said Bondoc "was a long-time friend and co-worker to many" and "our heartfelt condolences are with his shipmates, family, and friends."

To his wife and children, he was the one always thinking about the future. He had planned to retire soon, his wife said.

Sitting under a small weathered American flag in the shade on her patio on a recent Friday, she teared up as she shared the words her 11-year-old daughter has been asking her:

"How are we going to live now?"

Inewsource intern Natallie Rocha contributed to this report

Jill Castellano and Mary Plummer
Uncounted: San Diego County's Pandemic Victims Far Surpass Official Totals

> *This story was originally produced and published by inewsource, a nonprofit, nonpartisan newsroom in San Diego committed to exposing wrongdoing and holding powerful people and institutions accountable. As part of their commitment to keeping the San Diego community informed, inewsource has allowed this story to be reprinted and shared here with you. To learn more about their work and how you can support their journalism, visit inewsource.org.*

October 21, 2020

A 22-year-old died of an apparent overdose on his birthday after getting furloughed.

An 81-year-old with a chronic health condition couldn't go to the gym and lost her life five months later.

A farmworker in a family of undocumented immigrants contracted COVID-19 but—too scared to share his personal information—was never tested.

None of them are captured in the county's official list of coronavirus deaths, but their families say all of them died because of the pandemic.

A review of state and county public health data finds many more people have died as a result of the pandemic than the San Diego County public health office has acknowledged publicly.

Estimates from an inewsource analysis show that roughly 1,181 more county residents have died from March through August than in a normal year. The number is 66% higher than the county's official COVID-19 death total during that time.

The uncounted deaths are concentrated in minority communities and inside residents' homes, inewsource found. More than a third of the people excluded from the county's death total are Hispanic, and deaths are increasing faster at home than in hospitals.

While the public health office's data only captures people who tested positive for COVID-19, inewsource's analysis is much broader. It includes people who died from the virus but were never tested, as well as those who didn't contract it but lost their lives because of the pandemic anyway.

The analysis is an estimate of what epidemiologists call excess deaths, or the rise in deaths beyond what's expected in a normal year, based on data since January 2017.

"Excess deaths mean the deaths that could have been avoided, potentially," said Mark Hayward, a mortality researcher at the University of Texas Austin.

"It's a blip," he added. "There's a cause here, and the cause is not getting the care that people need."

In an email, a spokesperson for the county's health agency, Sarah Sweeney, said the analysis was "premature" and should not be conducted until after the pandemic is over, if at all.

Another staff member from the agency also questioned the findings, saying this kind of calculation should be used after floods or wildfires rather than during pandemics.

Andrew Noymer, an epidemiologist at UC Irvine who studies pandemic diseases, disagreed.

"That is absolutely wrong," said Noymer, after learning of the county's position. He has worked on excess deaths calculations in Orange County during COVID-19.

Experts have encouraged using this measurement during the COVID-19 crisis, and the Centers for Disease Control and Prevention has a regularly updating dashboard with excess deaths estimates for each state. Researchers have performed these calculations throughout pandemics since as far back as 1847 during London's flu outbreak.

Inewsource consulted with eight epidemiologists and mortality researchers who supported calculating excess deaths during COVID-19. They acknowledged that the estimates will become more accurate further into the pandemic because the data is still preliminary, but they said it's still important to make the public aware of the early findings now.

Dr. Matthew Wynia, the director of a bioethics program at the University of Colorado, said the official count kept by the public health office is important, but it "leads us to underestimate the total impact of certain types of disasters."

In September, Wynia and a team of researchers published a national report that Congress commissioned on how to measure a disaster's death toll. The report says an accurate picture of coronavirus deaths can have major effects on how governments allocate resources, including disaster relief money.

"You can use that information to target resources to neighborhoods that are being very hard hit or other social groups that may be particularly hard hit," Wynia said.

"When we can figure out why people die, we can maybe intervene to prevent those deaths," he added.

Reaching the Hardest Hit

Nancy Maldonado didn't need to see the numbers to know they were true.

As the CEO of the Chicano Federation, Maldonado had spoken with Latino residents in San Diego County for months who felt discouraged from seeking COVID-19 tests. Some worried about the stigma around testing positive, some didn't believe the healthcare system would help them, and others feared handing over personal information.

The rise in deaths during the pandemic bears out the consequences of those concerns. Hispanics—and other racial and ethnic minorities—are underrepresented in the county's official COVID-19 death total, which only includes people with positive tests.

About 55% more Hispanic residents are captured in inewsource's death data than in the county's. Plus, there are more than twice as many Asian people and Black people in the excess deaths data than are captured in the county's numbers.

"Honestly, it's not surprising," Maldonado said about the results.

"This isn't the equalizer," she added. "This isn't happening the same to everybody. We're not all in this together."

When someone gets tested for the virus, that information is reported to the county public health office, where the data is aggregated, stripped of identifiable information like name and birthday, and then released online to keep the public informed of the pandemic's impact in the region.

Maldonado said undocumented immigrants are especially concerned about entering their personal information into this system, even though officials have said they won't turn it over to law enforcement agencies.

In August, Maldonado asked an undocumented family if they would be willing to publicly talk about their father, a farmworker on a work visa who they believe contracted the virus from his co-workers in the fields. He died after developing COVID-19 symptoms, but he was never tested for the virus.

She told the family that sharing the full story could help prevent similar situations in the future. The family declined, fearing it would risk their safety.

"They lost their father, and they can't even talk about it because they're so scared," Maldonado said.

Roughly 1 in 20 county residents are undocumented immigrants, according to a recent estimate, surpassing the national average.

"There's no way we're not undercounting folks who are undocumented, folks who are migrant workers, folks who live in mixed-status households," said Rebecca Fielding-Miller, an assistant professor of public health at UC San Diego.

Fielding-Miller partnered with the Chicano Federation to interview Latinos about the county's contact tracing program, which tracks down people who may have COVID-19 and encourages them to self-isolate and get tested. They learned that language and cultural barriers discouraged Latino residents from participating.

Now, the Chicano Federation has a county-funded $2.6 million grant to continue pandemic-related outreach and education in the region's hardest-hit neighborhoods.

"I'm glad that it's being addressed, but it's unfortunate that it took so long," Maldonado said.

National researchers have found a magnifying effect of every COVID-19 death. They estimate each victim leaves behind nine grieving loved ones who are more likely to develop chronic mental illnesses or substance abuse disorders if they don't receive proper support.

About 180 more local Hispanic residents died as a result of the pandemic than are captured in the county's official data. That's more than 1,600 grieving family members who could benefit from support programs or nonprofit outreach.

"We need to know how big an effect this disease is having in our community," Fielding-Miller said.

"To say that somebody's uncle, somebody's grandmother, somebody's cousin, was a part of this historic pandemic and witnessing that is also a really important thing to be able to do."

Testing the System

In San Diego County, deaths at home continue to rise while deaths at hospitals have mostly stayed flat.

"I think a certain degree of it is people's fear of going to the hospital and getting the virus," said Dr. Steven Woolf, director emeritus at the Center on Society and Health at Virginia Commonwealth University. His recent study found 225,000 excess deaths across the country during the pandemic.

"The other issue is the virus itself," Woolf added. "It is a lethal virus, and for many patients the clinical progression is very fast."

That means some people don't make it to a healthcare clinic for testing before becoming isolated at home. And if they never visit a hospital, where COVID-19 testing is common, it's another missed opportunity to detect the virus.

"If a patient dies of a cardiac arrest, you don't know exactly what the struggle was," Woolf said. "The family members may say they were having trouble breathing for the last couple of days. Was that COVID? Was that congestive heart failure?"

The county's public health office has systems to identify these residents—the ones who died from a COVID-19 infection without a positive test—but the systems are limited.

For one, the county follows guidance from the National Center for Health Statistics on filling out death certificates during the pandemic. If someone likely had the virus but no test to confirm it, the paperwork should note that COVID-19 was "probable" or "presumed."

While some jurisdictions like New York City publicly release these probable death numbers, San Diego County does not. Inewsource found at least one resident whose death certificate listed COVID-19 as the cause but was not included in the county's numbers because the person didn't have a positive test on record.

Sweeney, the county spokesperson, said the public health office tracks probable deaths and is still working with the state to finalize the data before releasing it.

In the meantime, the county Medical Examiner's Office can take a probable case of COVID-19 and confirm it by testing a body for the virus. If it's positive, the county can add that information to a death certificate and include the COVID-19 victim in its official data.

The office tested at least 72 people who died at home from March through August, and four of them were positive. Hayward, the epidemiologist at UT Austin, reviewed the office's testing criteria and said it was robust, especially compared to rural areas of the U.S.

However, most people don't end up at the county morgue. The Medical Examiner's Office began about 1,600 death investigations from March 1 to August 5, a period when about 10,000 residents died.

County officials have acknowledged their death totals have failed to capture all those who died from the coronavirus, but they've said their data has gotten better as testing has become more widespread.

"I think it may be that there were some deaths that occurred early on during the pandemic, say in March and April, that may have been due to COVID but not attributed to COVID," said Dr. Eric McDonald, the county's medical director of epidemiology and immunization services. "But I think that that is not really a problem going forward."

"He Was My Person"

The coronavirus has taken the lives of San Diego County residents who never contracted it, but mortality data can't explain what exactly was responsible for their deaths.

"That kind of information just isn't available," said David Leon, an epidemiologist at the London School of Hygiene & Tropical Medicine who co-authored a paper on excess deaths during the pandemic.

The answers would have to come from "qualitative research," he said, like interviews with the loved ones of those who died.

"I think the question of how one gets to the bottom of that is very difficult.... It would involve going to talk to family doctors and perhaps people who've lost relatives," Leon said.

The mother of Zach Budlong, a Vista resident, believes her son is one of the county's indirect victims.

Zach left the world on August 23, the same day he came into it. It was his 22nd birthday.

When the pandemic struck, he was helping care for his sister as she neared the end of high school, enjoying his work and surfing regularly with a group of close friends.

Then Zach was furloughed from his job at Caliber Collision, and he lost routine and structure, his mom said. He spent more time with friends and drank more alcohol than he had before.

With no work, he worried about the future, and when federal unemployment benefits were cut from $600 to $200 a week, his anxiety grew. Paying rent became a struggle.

"He was just worried. It's expensive," said Zach's mother, Rachel Budlong, who lives in Austin, Texas. "It's a lot of stress to live out there and to not be able to make money."

Zach also started to look up conspiracy theories about COVID-19.

"I think he just thought COVID wasn't real, he was invincible, nothing bad was going to happen to him because nothing bad had ever happened to his friends," his mom said. "And that's what scares me."

On the Saturday of his birthday weekend, Zach went to the beach and a friend's barbecue to celebrate. The partying carried into the next day. Friends and family suspect it was at some point early Sunday that he unknowingly took fentanyl, a synthetic opioid, thinking it was Xanax.

His girlfriend, Sierra Weirich, walked over from her nearby home around 7 AM to check on him. When she found Zach, he was unconscious. His roommate, a friend and an acquaintance were in the apartment.

Weirich screamed, called 911 and went for help. A nurse walking her two dogs nearby rushed in and administered CPR. The police and paramedics arrived, but no one could resuscitate him.

"He was my person," said Weirich, 20, who first met Zach in middle school. He was a "pure soul," she said, had a "contagious laugh," and "wanted good for everyone."

"This is not how life was supposed to go."

Zach died shortly after sunrise from a presumed drug overdose. The toxicology report is still pending, his mother said.

He leaves behind his parents, his 17-year-old sister, Casey, and his 25-year-old brother, Jacob. His mother said the pandemic impacted the whole family, but no one more than Zach.

"He had nothing to do and so much time on his hands and with anxiety," she said, her voice trailing off.

Ultimately, she said, it led to a toxic environment.

"That's why I think the pandemic played such a part in his death. And I'm afraid, I'm afraid for his friends. I'm afraid for any kids that are in a similar position," she said.

"I think that a lot of young people are struggling right now."

The virus itself isn't a major health risk to younger people—there were only three reported COVID-19 deaths among county residents in their 20s through August—but the pandemic has caused them harm in other ways.

That age group accounts for about 100 excess deaths in the first six months of the pandemic.

McDonald, who oversees the county's epidemiology and immunizations services, said the region's rise in deaths beyond those with COVID-19 infections is "an issue that's been on the mind of both the public and healthcare providers."

"We will have to look into that, and we are looking into that actively," he said.

Homebound

When a major hurricane makes landfall, only a fraction of the victims die from the high winds and flooding. Some freeze in their homes when the power goes out, slowly suffer from starvation, or develop carbon monoxide poisoning from their backup generators. These are the disaster's indirect deaths.

In the case of COVID-19, the common example used by researchers of an indirect death is people too scared to go to a hospital, fearing they may catch the virus, who die at home from a heart attack.

But deaths during the pandemic come from many—and sometimes unexpected—causes.

The brother of Steve Hoen, a 55-year-old who lived near Pacific Beach, said the pandemic forced Steve into a sedentary lifestyle that led to his death.

Steve was a free-spirited athlete who loved the outdoors and gravitated toward the ocean. Between golf, surfing, boxing and jiu jitsu, he always found a way to stay active. But the avid athlete was born with a heart defect, even though it wasn't easy to tell, and took blood thinners his whole life to avoid dangerous clots.

His brother, Paul Hoen, said he managed it well—in fact, he was in "perfect health"—until the pandemic, when his usual surf spots shut down, the gyms closed, and he was instructed to work from home.

Steve died from a blood clot in his heart on May 4, leaving behind his father, brother, and sister.

"It upends the whole rhythm of a person's life," Paul Hoen said about the pandemic. "And for a person who required his blood clotting levels to be at a certain level, suddenly upending the normal I think is dangerous."

Rosie Sanchez, an 81-year-old Lakeside resident, was a prolific gym-goer, too.

It was a habit she developed after polio almost took her at age 12, when her muscles atrophied and she was unable to walk for three years.

Rosie's daughter, Becky McBride, said her mom's workout routine prevented her muscles from atrophying, which can happen to former polio patients as they age. In March, Rosie still coached two softball teams from her wheelchair, lived independently with her cousin, and went to the gym every day.

But when gyms were forced to close, her routine turned upside down. Rosie, a devoted Padres fan and season ticket holder since 1978 who also traveled regularly to NASCAR races, was suddenly homebound.

By May, Rosie couldn't stand. She lost so much muscle in her legs and torso that she couldn't hold her head up or reposition herself without help.

"She kept saying, 'Everything's falling apart. Everything's falling apart,'" McBride said. "She never talks like that. And I thought, what is she talking about? But she couldn't see her softball teams. She couldn't go to her sporting events. She couldn't see her family, really. So it was very hard to not be depressed."

Following a hospitalization, Rosie died at home on August 11.

Her daughter said she regrets that she didn't get her mom a personal trainer during the state-ordered shutdown, but she expected the gyms would open up soon and her mom would recover.

"I guess I just wish we could have lived our lives and made our own choices," McBride said.

"This is all so unnatural."

Inewsource intern Sofía Mejías-Pascoe contributed to this story

Will Huntsberry

The First Year of COVID: Farm and Construction Workers Among Those Most Likely to Die

This story was first published by Voice of San Diego.

December 16, 2021

Robert Mejia was recently visited by a certain kind of grief. It was both the absence and presence of his father.

Robert, who is 24, was sitting in the bleachers watching his younger brother play high school basketball—a role his dad used to fill. Jayme, their father, used to yell a lot from the bench.

As Robert sat there trying to fill that role, thinking of all the things Jayme might have said, he suddenly felt overwhelmed by the sense that his dad was there.

"I was in parent mode, watching, and I just started crying because I wish my dad was here to see this," said Robert. "I could literally feel him."

Robert and his seven brothers and sisters are about to face their first Christmas without their father. Jayme died alone in a hospital last January from complications related to COVID-19. He was 43 years old.

His family isn't quite sure where he caught COVID, but one possibility is his job site. Jayme was a heavy equipment operator in the construction industry—a profession overrepresented among those who died, according to a new analysis of death certificates by Voice of San Diego.

As part of an ongoing series, Year One: COVID-19's Death Toll, a team of reporters logged more than 4,000 death certificates—one for each COVID-related death during the first year of the pandemic. COVID-19 is far more deadly for elders, but more than 1,000 people who died were 65 or younger.

Voice of San Diego categorized the professions of each of those working-age San Diegans, according to U.S. Census industry codes. The analysis reveals that COVID ripped through some working-class professions, even as white-collar professionals tended to be more isolated.

Agricultural workers were hit harder than any other group. Their share of the death toll was 612 percent higher than their share of San Diego County's workers.

A wide-ranging Census category that encompasses security guards, custodians, and clerical workers experienced the second most disparate death rate.

Construction workers had the third highest death rate—and represented the single highest number of deaths. Out of 1,024 working-age people who died, 132 worked in construction.

"It's sad. It's an unfortunate thing," said Kelvin Barrios, community engagement director of the Laborers Local Union 89, which represents nearly 4,000 construction workers in San Diego.

Barrios, however, was quick to point out that no working-age members of Local 89 died from COVID-19. He said the union went above and beyond state guidelines in creating safety protocols for job sites.

It's unclear exactly why construction workers died at such high rates.

Robert said his dad Jayme, who had diabetes, was always extra careful about washing his hands and trying to keep his distance. But Jayme told him that fellow workers frequently showed up to work with a cough and that it wasn't exactly easy to wash his hands on job sites.

Ricardo Favela is the son of a farmworker and grew up in Fallbrook, which calls itself the avocado capital of the world. He volunteers with a group called Voces de Fallbrook that does advocacy and outreach for farmworkers.

"In town we know many wives that are widowed, brothers that have been lost, parents. It's hit this community pretty hard," he said.

Life for farm workers can be "very secluded," said Favela. That means farmworkers have had less access to good information, healthcare facilities, COVID tests and now the vaccine.

Better outreach to farmworkers, Favela said, could have led to better outcomes. He pointed to a recent vaccine drive to illustrate his point.

Volunteers in Fallbrook started knocking on doors a few weeks ago to tell people about a free vaccine clinic. The door-to-door campaign led to 200 people being vaccinated. Getting information and services to rural communities, said Favela, requires this kind of boots-on-the-ground approach.

"The irony that I don't think we've come to terms within this community is that the workers that produce this fruit we're so proud of are relegated to margins of society here," he said.

Favela also mentioned that many farmworkers live in multi-generational housing, which means COVID could have been spread between family members living in the same house.

Some trends previously revealed by Voice were even more pronounced among working-age people. For instance, 60 percent of working-age San Diegans who died were immigrants. The same was true for 52 percent of all people who died. Among working-age people, 65 percent who died were Latino—even though Latinos represented 53 percent of all deaths.

Income also seems to be linked to death rates. Lower-income ZIP codes had significantly higher rates of death. In fact, for every $6,600 increase in median income, death rates went down by ten percent.

Among the four industries with significantly elevated risk of death—which include farmworkers, custodians and landscapers, construction workers and transportation workers—none have a median income higher than $50,000 per year.

The professions with significantly decreased rates of death aren't a surprise.

Professional service providers like lawyers, accountants, and architects were the least likely working-age San Diegans to die. They represent nearly 11 percent of the population, but less than one percent of all deaths.

Finance workers and real estate professionals also had significantly decreased rates of death. Interestingly, people working in retail shops like grocery stores or shoe stores also had decreased rates of death, despite many of them remaining essential during the pandemic.

Education workers, such as teachers, also had decreased rates of death.

Maria Rosario Araneta, a public health professor at UC San Diego, said the findings are consistent with research into excess deaths during the pandemic. Food and agriculture workers were among those with the highest excess death rates.

An excess death analysis shows the number of people who died by any cause compared to all deaths in a typical year. Voice's analysis specifically measured those who died related to COVID.

Robert and his mom and brothers and sisters are left trying to rebuild a life they thought would include their father for many more years to come. Jayme was the person they all went to for advice or to be picked up when they were down.

"I don't think we all show it too much to each other, but it's really hard," said Robert. "I don't understand life anymore."

Bella Ross contributed to this report

MacKenzie Elmer

Volunteers Take Vaccine Appointments Door to Door in Barrio Logan

This story was first published by Voice of San Diego.

April 5, 2021

Governor Gavin Newsom recently praised San Diego both for getting as many vaccines in arms as it has and for reaching communities hit hardest by the pandemic, calling the city a state leader in vaccinating equity.

But that means the rest of the state's communities of color are still in dire need of a life-saving vaccine.

"The rich and the powerful tend to be first in line," said Christian Ramers, an infectious disease specialist at San Diego State University who oversees clinical programs at Family Health Centers of San Diego.

And the rich and the powerful tend to be White. That inequity is starkly apparent in vaccine data kept by San Diego County.

As of March 30, 48 percent of San Diegans 16 and older who got at least one dose of the vaccine are White. Twenty percent are Hispanic or Latino. The county's population is 45 percent White. But 34 percent identify as Hispanic or Latino.

While Whites are getting vaccines the fastest, "they need it the least," Ramers said.

Latinos are resoundingly suffering the most with 120,000 positive COVID-19 cases in San Diego County. Whites have about 60,000 cases. More Latinos have died from COVID-19 than any other racial or ethnic group.

Ramers said it takes extra effort to reach them, though. There's deep-seated suspicion of government in these communities like Barrio Logan and Logan Heights, where the federal government has severed the neighborhoods with interstate highways, among a litany of other historic policy decisions that disenfranchise non-White populations.

Ramers said while mass vaccination sites, like the superstations at the Grossmont Center mall and a former Sears in Chula Vista, work well for getting as many shots in arms as possible, the "Hunger Games" approach actually drives disparity. Those sites tend to favor those who are more nimble with the internet and have resources to drive over a dozen miles to reach an unfilled appointment at a moment's notice.

"What it takes to avoid that is a shoe-level, door-to-door campaign, and keeping others from swooping in and taking the slots," Ramers said.

And that's precisely what Barrio Logan did last week.

Thanks to a change in tactic by President Joe Biden's administration, the federal government started sending more vaccines directly to federally funded clinics like Family Health Centers of San Diego. In anticipation of a 2,000-vaccine shipment Saturday, the community wrangled groups of volunteers to knock on doors and sign up as many people living in or near the 92113 ZIP code as possible.

The center has a vaccination site set up in its parking lot, where anyone with an appointment can get one. But "a lot of people outside the neighborhood were taking them," Anthony White, the center's director of community and government relations, told the Barrio Logan Community Planning Group during a March meeting.

In just an hour of door-knocking on Wednesday, volunteers Soraya Morales and Marcela Mercado reached over a dozen residents at their doorsteps, including elderly residents who didn't even know the vaccine was available.

That included 62-year-old Marta Barraza. As of March 15, she was eligible to get a vaccine but thought they were still only reserved for doctors, nurses, and teachers—who, she argued, should have them before herself.

Many things about the pandemic brought her to tears as she stood on her porch, giving the volunteer her information for an appointment.

The locked doors at Church of the Immaculate Conception in Old Town hurt her the most.

"I had a couple of things to say to God, but I couldn't. So I was looking up at the sky to talk to him," Barraza said, reflecting on the pandemic year.

The church doors finally opened that Wednesday, and Barraza, wearing a mask, was able to go to mass.

"I wanted to go to the altar, where we have a big figure of Jesus, and hold him; that's how happy I was to see him," she said.

David Alvarez, a former San Diego city councilman from the neighborhood, helped organize the door-knockers.

"This area has been the hardest hit and falling behind on vaccination," Alvarez told about 10 volunteers on Wednesday.

He pushed them to get phone numbers and names of potential patients to secure a spot in line. The health center reserved a special phone line for neighborhood patients so residents, especially elderly ones, didn't have to use a computer to sign up.

It was successful, he said. After four days of campaigning, volunteers visited over 4,000 houses and registered a quarter of them.

Morales and Mercado signed up grandmothers for appointments through the gates of their homes or as they carted groceries down the street. Mercado reached Deysi Solis as she was leaving her house with her two children.

"I was positive for COVID earlier in the year," Solis said. "We wanted a vaccine, but we heard there weren't any."

Maya Srikrishnan
The First Year of COVID: Filipinos Were Among Hardest Hit, But Hidden by Data

This story was first published by Voice of San Diego.

December 6, 2021

The day after Christmas, Glenda Monzon, her husband Rey Monzon, and their son discovered they had been exposed to COVID-19.

Glenda and her son tested positive, but her husband tested negative. Her son quarantined in his apartment in Ventura County, and Glenda quarantined downstairs in her house, trying to stay away from her husband and sanitize everything she touched. They told their daughter, who had been staying with them but had been away for the holidays, to stay away.

But it became clear that something was wrong with Rey. He started developing back pains. Rey was tested again and again—each time his test came back negative.

After a few days, he went to the doctor. They tested him three times before one showed him positive for COVID.

On January 7, Glenda's son texted her in the morning to tell her he couldn't breathe and drove himself to the emergency room. Thirty minutes later, Rey went upstairs and said he couldn't breathe. She took him to the hospital.

Because Glenda was also positive, she couldn't stay. For several days, she received updates from doctors about both her son and husband, who seemed to be going through the same treatment. Her son started to get better and would soon be released—though with oxygen—but Rey kept getting worse.

His kidneys were starting to fail, so doctors put him on dialysis and upped his medication. On January 21, he was placed on a ventilator.

"They didn't think he was going to make it," Glenda said. Her sister picked up Glenda's son, who was still on oxygen and couldn't drive, to bring him home.

At 2:30 a.m. on January 23, she got a call that they should go see Rey. Only two people would be allowed inside the hospital to see him—and it would still be through glass. She and her son had a half hour, while their daughter and other family members waited in the parking lot. They said goodbye over FaceTime.

He passed away soon after at Scripps Green Hospital.

"It can hit you and you don't even know it," Glenda said.

Rey was 63, but healthy. He had high blood pressure but ran two miles every morning. He had been an advocate and leader in the Filipino community his whole life.

When he was a student at San Diego State University, he wrote his thesis and dissertation on Filipino college students and family relations. Monzon turned that into a career, working at San Diego State in research and data, but also helping to guide Filipino students as they made their way through school.

Filipinos were among the hardest-hit communities by COVID-19 in San Diego County—but that cost was largely hidden because the county reported cases and deaths among Filipinos within a broad category of Asian Americans, rather than breaking them out specifically. A Voice of San Diego analysis of death certificates of everyone who died from COVID-19 in the first year of the pandemic in San Diego County, though, shows the disparate impact the virus had on the region's Filipino community.

Filipinos accounted for about 7 percent of the 4,000 COVID-19 deaths during the pandemic's first year, while they make up roughly 6.5 percent of the county population. That made Filipinos the third largest nationality for pandemic deaths in the county during that time.

But that disparity still understates the toll the virus took on the Filipino community. Dr. Maria Rosario Araneta, a professor of family medicine and public health at UC San Diego School of Medicine, argued that looking at deaths per 100,000 people better reflects the effects the virus had on smaller populations, like Filipinos.

In that analysis, Filipinos had the second highest mortality rate in the county during the pandemic's first year. The Filipino mortality rate was 120 deaths per 100,000 people. That's lower than the Latino mortality rate of 170 per 100,000, but far higher than the White mortality rate of roughly 38 per 100,000. Looking at the death rate per 100,000, Araneta said, is a common way of looking at populations of different sizes to determine who is most at risk.

Filipinos faced a unique set of risks. Many Filipinos work in the health care sector or in other essential, high-risk employment, like in assisted living facilities. They also tend to live in multigenerational households and suffer from certain health conditions that increase morbidity with COVID, like diabetes and hypertension. The majority of Filipinos who died, 92 percent, were immigrants, while only 8 percent were U.S.-born.

But because Filipino deaths and cases weren't specifically tracked by the county—grouped instead with other Asian nationalities, which had lower numbers of cases and deaths—community advocates and researchers said that the community didn't get the support and resources it needed.

A Unique Set of Risks

Filipinos make up nearly a fifth of registered nurses in California, according to a 2018 Board of Registered Nursing survey. Soon after the Philippines became a U.S. colony in 1898, the United States implemented American nursing programs there. In the 1960s, a change in U.S. immigration laws and a shortage of nurses resulted in many Filipino nurses coming to the United States to work.

Their prevalence in health care jobs—and the risk it puts them at to contract COVID-19—is clear.

According to the death certificates analyzed by VOSD in which occupation was reported, 14.6 percent of Filipinos who died were health care workers, while health care workers represented just 6.2 percent of non-Filipino pandemic deaths.

It's even more stark among the working-age population. Among those 65 years old and younger, 20 percent of Filipinos who died were health care workers compared to 6 percent among non-Filipino deaths. Almost one-fourth of Filipino COVID deaths were people under 65.

This reflected a nationwide trend. A September 2020 report from National Nurses United, the country's largest nursing union, found that even though Filipino nurses make up only 4 percent of the nursing population nationwide, nearly a third of nurses who have died from the coronavirus in the country are Filipino.

It is not clear why Filipino nurses and healthcare workers seemed to have been more impacted than healthcare workers of other ethnicities.

And while education level was a determinant for who lived and died from COVID throughout the county, Filipinos were an outlier, likely because of their prevalence in the healthcare industry. A college education didn't offer protection from COVID deaths for many Filipinos. Although only 17 percent of people who died from COVID between March 2020 and March 2021 had a bachelor's degree, among Filipinos who died from COVID in that time period, 34.5 percent had a bachelor's degree.

In December, Gemma Rama-Banaag remembers coming home from work as Chief Nursing Officer at Paradise Valley Hospital with a terrible headache. She napped while her husband, Dr. Chester Banaag, made dinner. That happened several nights in a row before her youngest son called to say he and his girlfriend, who both work in hospitals, were showing symptoms of COVID-19. The family had been spending time together. All four tested positive.

"My first concern was my husband because he was the highest risk," Rama-Banaag said.

Banaag retired from his dentistry practice in 2016, when he was 53 years old. He spent his years in retirement involved in community activities—from becoming the West Coast ambassador by the USA Pickleball Association and founding the first pickleball park in Chula Vista to participating in medical-dental missions to Tijuana to being an active youth mentor in his church community.

A few days later, they went to the hospital because Banaag was looking weak. His oxygen saturation was low, and he was placed in the ICU. A few days later Rama-Banaag took a turn for the worse and was also admitted to the hospital for two nights.

By the time Rama-Banaag got home, the kids had recovered. Banaag also seemed to be doing better. But then suddenly, he had to be intubated a few days later.

Everything had been improving, except Banaag's lungs, Rama-Banaag said. They knew his last chance would be an extracorporeal membrane oxygenation, and called around the state for an ECMO machine, something in high demand during the 2020 holidays, when COVID cases surged statewide.

A childhood friend of Rama-Banaag's was an ECMO nurse at St. John's Well Child and Family Center in Los Angeles. The family flew him there, but the treatment didn't work.

"By that time, we knew he wasn't going to make it," Rama-Banaag said. She was still weak from COVID but stayed at a hotel close by, so she and her family could be with him.

On January 1, 2021, Banaag died from COVID-19.

A report from the UC Davis Bulosan Center for Filipinx Studies found Filipinos were an at-risk group during the pandemic not only because of their exposure as health care workers but also economic insecurity, pre-existing health conditions, a lack of health insurance, and the fact that there are tens of thousands of undocumented Filipinos in California.

Rama-Banaag said Filipinos also have high rates of several health conditions that made it more likely to die from COVID. Her husband had hypertension, though it was well managed.

For example, one 2017 study found that Filipino Americans over 50 are at higher risk for diabetes—even if they're not obese—when compared to their White counterparts. Another 2014 study found that hypertension among Filipino immigrants in the U.S. was disproportionately high when compared to other Asian groups and to Whites.

The Data Problem

Rey Monzon was someone who was constantly trying to bring data and research about the experiences of Filipinos to the forefront, said JoAnn Fields, a Filipino community advocate.

"Our community took a great loss when he passed," Fields said. "Who was working under him? Who had his research? COVID-19 showed again how people tried to erase us."

While the pandemic's toll on other groups, like Latinos, has been widely reported, its impact on Filipinos wasn't, because of the way deaths and cases were reported by public officials.

This mostly stemmed from the way data was collected and analyzed federally and at the state and county level.

Filipino advocates, medical professionals, and political leaders have long been calling for data that breaks down the Asian racial and ethnic category into subgroups based on different nationalities.

"We were screaming, 'disaggregate the data, disaggregate the data,' after the first couple of months of the pandemic," said Dr. GilAnthony Ungab, the CEO of the Southern California Center for Inclusion and Diversity. "Why didn't they do it?"

San Diego Mayor Todd Gloria, then in the state Assembly, sent a letter to Governor Gavin Newsom in August 2020, requesting that the California Department of Public Health report ethnicity by Asian subgroups "instead of using 'Asian American' as an overarching label."

In a statement, county spokeswoman Sarah Sweeney said the county didn't disaggregate the data because it uses categories set by the California Department of Public Health and the Centers for Disease Control and Prevention.

"These entities use this data to make funding and other prioritization decisions," Sweeney wrote. "Additionally, the hospital systems statewide do not include these categories in the information reported to us. In essence, the varied entities tracking and gathering this information all need to use the same standards and categories."

A handful of other jurisdictions, though, chose to disaggregate their data, revealing disparities.

Santa Clara County disaggregated its Asian coronavirus cases into subgroups and found Filipinos and Vietnamese people were being disproportionately impacted by the virus. Though Filipino Americans make up 13 percent of the Asian American population in the county, they accounted for 21 percent of coronavirus cases between June 1 and December 3 last year.

Hawaii has been disaggregating its data and found early on that the state's Filipino community had the second worst disparity in the state, making up 16 percent of the population but more than a fifth of confirmed coronavirus cases.

Voice of San Diego's death certificate analysis showed Filipinos made up more than 60 percent of all Asian deaths in the first year of the pandemic.

But there have been other ways COVID data has been presented that has hidden the risk for some populations, said Araneta, the UC San Diego School of Medicine professor of family medicine and public health.

For example, COVID-19 case-fatality rates—the proportion of people with COVID-19 who die from COVID-19—show Asians have been more likely to die from COVID once infected since the beginning of the pandemic.

In July 2020, the case-fatality rate among all San Diego COVID cases was 2 percent—meaning 2 percent of all San Diego COVID cases died. Among San Diego Asian COVID cases, though, that number rose to 5 percent. As of November 24, 1.1 percent of all San Diego COVID cases died, but 2.1 percent of Asian San Diego COVID cases died.

"When we realized the case-fatality rate for Asians was so high, we were concerned that maybe they weren't going to get tested because of the anti-Asian violence," Araneta said.

But clear data on specific communities is vital, Araneta, Ungab and Fields all said, because it determined which populations got funding for outreach, education, research, and other resources. As a result, organizations that specifically wanted to contact or research the Filipino community had less opportunity for county, state, or other funding.

"Unless you could demonstrate, especially in grant applications, that your community was at risk, then the perception was that your community wasn't in need," Araneta said. "It made it hard to do basic interventions such as public health messaging."

Funding could have been used to do more outreach, so Filipino health care workers living in multigenerational households could have safely isolated from the rest of their family, she said. There could have been efforts to look into whether there were reasons why Filipinos may not have been utilizing resources like the county hotel rooms that were offered.

"There's been an urgency with COVID, but the importance and calls for disaggregation preceded the pandemic," Araneta said. "California has the largest Asian American population in the country. It's important and necessary to understand the differences in the prevalence of certain conditions and the treatment."

Fields and Ungab started the San Diego Filipino COVID-19 Task Force shortly after the pandemic began in an effort to do outreach and education specific to the needs and risks of the community. But they said the effort has been completely unfunded.

"We do Zoom conferences," Ungab said. "JoAnn has been begging people to let us use their Zoom."

Sweeney said the county did give funds to groups that included the Filipino community in their outreach, the Union of Pan Asian Communities for outreach and education and Communities Fight COVID for contact tracing. UPAC received a $469,200 contract for September 2020 to December 2021 of millions that the county doled out during the pandemic for COVID-19-related health disparities and equity issues.

Fields said that wasn't sufficient. UPAC is only one organization and serves all Asian communities. She thinks governments haven't been concerned with helping the Filipino community.

"I know what's possible if there is political will, but now it seems like no one is willing to move for us," she said.

Maya Srikrishnan
Filipino Residents Have Been Hit Hard by COVID—But No One Knows Just How Hard

This story was first published by Voice of San Diego.

February 1, 2021

JoAnn Fields watched the funerals of two dear friends and leaders in the Filipino community in the last week of January. She has another memorial on the first day of February.

Since January 1, at least four men in her community have died of COVID-19.

On the first day of the year was Dr. Chester Banaag, a dentist and active member of the San Diego Filipino American Seventh Adventist church. Then, was Benjamin Clanor, who worked on audio during the Island Vibe Music Festival and other major events. Then there was Obie Sibug, a popular contractor in the community, and Rey Monzon, a researcher and faculty member at San Diego State who was an active supporter of Filipino and other Asian and Pacific Islander students.

"I'm talking to my friends and there are whole families who are COVID-19 positive," Field said. "Even in just my immediate family, I have cousins who are scared to be around their moms because they are nurses. This has not happened in our community before."

Filipino community leaders and health care workers in San Diego believe that their community has been hit especially hard by COVID-19, but data about the virus's impact specifically on Filipinos has proven hard to come by.

"I'm trying to direct my anger and sadness into advocacy," Fields said. "These people can't have died in vain."

Most public health data regarding the pandemic groups dozens of nationalities, who speak hundreds of different languages, under one category when it comes to race and ethnicity: "Asian." But not all Asian communities have been equally affected by the virus, and many in the Filipino community believe that being grouped with other communities may be hiding the true impact on Filipinos.

"What's critical, particularly in pandemics and epidemics, is you need to be able to communicate with at-risk communities," said Dr. Maria Rosario Araneta, a professor of family medicine and public health at UC San Diego School of Medicine.

There are several reasons why those in the Filipino community in San Diego believe they've been contracting and dying from COVID-19 at higher rates.

One is that some of the most affected ZIP codes in the county are also where Filipinos live.

"When I review the areas that have the highest number of cases, they are places with Filipinos," said Fields. "At one point it was 92154, where I was raised. Then there is 91910 in Chula Vista, where I live now, and 91950, which is National City, where we shop, where many Filipino businesses are."

Mira Mesa, which also has many Filipino residents, has also seen higher COVID infection rates than the communities surrounding it.

Many Filipinos work in the health care sector or in other essential, high-risk employment, like in assisted living facilities.

Filipinos make up nearly a fifth of registered nurses in California, according to a 2018 Board of Registered Nursing survey. Soon after the Philippines became a U.S. colony in 1898, the United States implemented American nursing programs in the country. Then in the 1960s, a change in U.S. immigration laws and a shortage of nurses resulted in many Filipino nurses coming to the United States to work.

"If we know the numbers a little bit better, then it's easier to start looking at the issue and try to figure out what is happening and why," said Crisamar Anunciado, a senior medical liaison for AstraZeneca.

What the Existing Data Shows

There is some limited data, both nationwide and from other localities, that show Filipinos have been hit harder than other groups.

A September 2020 report from National Nurses United, the country's largest nursing union, found that even though Filipino nurses make up only 4 percent of the nursing population nationwide, nearly a third of nurses who have died from the coronavirus in the country are Filipino.

Santa Clara County disaggregated its Asian coronavirus cases into subgroups and found that Filipinos and Vietnamese people were being disproportionately impacted by the virus. Though Filipino Americans make up 13 percent of the Asian American population in the county, they accounted for 21 percent of coronavirus cases between June 1 and December 3 last year.

Data collected by the *Los Angeles Times* in July 2020 found that Filipino Americans accounted for at least 35 percent of coronavirus deaths among Asians in California. The *Times* also reported at the time that of 48 Filipino Americans known by the Philippine Consulate General of Los Angeles to have been infected with the coronavirus, 19 had died. Though that data is very limited, it suggests a 40 percent mortality rate—far higher than the overall mortality rate from the virus.

There are 43 contact tracers working for San Diego County or county contractors who speak Tagalog, according to county spokeswoman Sarah Sweeney. Four of those also speak Ilocano, another language spoken by some in the Philippines. Sweeney said that since May 5, 2020,

0.7 percent of individuals interviewed by contact tracers requested to be interviewed in Tagalog. This is also likely an underestimate of Filipino cases, since many speak English.

Data locally wasn't disaggregated from the state largely because at the federal level, all Asian subgroups are categorized as one, said Araneta. But that doesn't mean states and counties can't choose to report their data in more detail. Hawaii, for example, has been disaggregating its data and it revealed that the state's Filipino community had the second worst disparity in the state, making up 16 percent of the population but more than a fifth of confirmed coronavirus cases.

Araneta said she received some data from the California Department of Health that showed case fatality rates—meaning how many people who have confirmed cases are dying—were high among Asians both statewide and in San Diego County. (Araneta said she wasn't able to share specific numbers with the media.)

"The message I want to convey is the urgency of disaggregation, especially in the state with the largest Asian American population," Araneta said. "It hinders our ability to provide information and resources to people. If we don't have information on subgroups, how do we know what languages to use to reach out to people in need and what venues to target? Do we go to Vietnamese temples or Filipino churches?"

The lack of data about Filipino deaths can also feed into misinformation about the pandemic and the vaccine, said Dr. GilAnthony Ungab, a cardiologist at Sharp Chula Vista and the founder of the Sharp Chula Vista Center for Inclusion and Diversity in Clinical Research.

"As doctors, it would be easier to get the community on board if we had data that showed that Filipino people were dying in San Diego," Ungab said.

A March report from the UC Davis Bulosan Center for Filipinx Studies found that Filipinos were an at-risk group during the pandemic because of not only their exposure as health care workers, but also because of economic insecurity, pre-existing health conditions, a lack of health insurance, and the fact that there are tens of thousands of undocumented Filipinos in California.

Araneta and Anunciado also pointed out that there are also other risk factors, like that Filipinos are more likely to live in multigenerational households.

San Diego County's Challenge

San Diego has one of the largest Filipino populations in the country.

Between 2014 and 2018, the San Diego–Carlsbad metropolitan region had the fourth largest immigrant population from the Philippines in the country, totaling about 98,000 people, according to the Migration Policy Institute. That makes up 3 percent of the region's population. The total Filipino population in the region, which also includes those born in the United States, is around 200,000. After Spanish, Tagalog is the second-most-spoken non-English language in the county.

So it would stand to reason, the Filipino advocates and health care workers Voice of San Diego spoke to agreed, that the data from elsewhere in the country showing COVID-19 hitting Filipinos especially hard would be relevant here.

"We are such a large ethnic group," Fields said. "But when we fall under this umbrella of [Asian American and Pacific Islander] that is so huge and diverse, it's really hard to voice concerns. It feels like our entire community is an afterthought."

Disaggregating data could potentially identify other groups within the Asian American and Pacific Islander community who may be infected or dying at higher rates but whose plight remains hidden because they are grouped with so many other nationalities that may have far different experiences during the pandemic.

For example, disaggregated data in New York City showed that South Asians and Chinese New Yorkers were among the racial and ethnic groups hardest hit by the pandemic.

But such data in San Diego County hasn't yet been made available, at least not publicly, though many in the community have been asking for it—and have even volunteered to do the work if the county would be willing to partner with them or provide some funds to do so.

"This is something we have been asking for a while now," said San Diego City Councilman Chris Cate, who is Filipino and represents Mira Mesa, which has a large number of Filipino residents. "I don't know what the issue is. We have a large Filipino community here in San Diego. Elected leaders and policy leaders need to recognize the community and its needs."

Cate said he worked to get a testing site in Mira Mesa to ensure people in the community have access to testing.

San Diego Mayor Todd Gloria also sent a letter to Governor Gavin Newsom in August, requesting that the California Department of Public Health report ethnicity by Asian subgroups "instead of using 'Asian American' as an overarching label."

The county did not respond to questions about why the data hasn't been broken down, but county spokeswoman Sweeney said people self-identify their race or ethnicity for the county's data collection.

"If you don't have the data that shows your community is in need, then when funds come that could help, they don't come to you," Fields said. "That is a form of racism."

That's why Fields, Ungab, and others started their own Filipino COVID-19 Task Force, to try to provide information and a voice for Filipinos throughout the pandemic. But even with community members and those in health care willing to take on the additional work, it's hard to get more specific data without the county's cooperation.

Other studies have used things like algorithms that analyze last names to divide past data into subgroups, and Ungab and Araneta think such analyses are possible to do in San Diego.

Ungab said he is hoping for a grant so that the Sharp Chula Vista Center for Inclusion and Diversity in Clinical Research could analyze and disaggregate the data. He said he did not receive a grant when they were previously given out by the county.

Araneta also said she has offered to do the disaggregation work for San Diego but hasn't received any response. On a brighter note, she did say she had several Tagalog-speaking medical students who were volunteering to work at the vaccine superstations in South Bay to help encourage more Filipinos in the community to get vaccinated.

Anunciado said she thinks the county is doing the best it can, but "what you don't see is what you don't see."

"Until we collect the data and have hard numbers, it's hard to start fixing what is wrong," she said.

Maya Srikrishnan
Coronavirus Hit Latinos Harder Thanks to a Perfect Storm of Disparities

This story was first published by Voice of San Diego.

August 12, 2020

Edith Abundis, a teacher at the Chicano Federation's Child Development Center, got a call from her uncle in early May. He wasn't feeling well.

A few days later, he was hospitalized with the coronavirus.

A few days after Abundis's uncle went to the hospital, her aunt followed.

Abundis's uncle passed away. He was 71 years old. Neither she nor her parents could attend the small funeral for fear of the virus.

Her aunt eventually recovered, was taken off a ventilator and is home, though she still needs oxygen. She didn't know her husband had died until roughly a month later, because she, too, was in the hospital, unable to see her family.

"My best friend's dad passed away from the virus, also," Abundis said. "Now I am just so fearful."

Abundis's experience is indicative of the pandemic's disproportionate impact on Latinos, who are more likely than other racial groups to contract, be hospitalized, and die from COVID-19.

Although they make up 34 percent of San Diego County's population, Latinos account for 62 percent of confirmed COVID-19 cases, 61 percent of hospitalizations and 45 percent of COVID deaths. The virus's disproportionate impact on Latinos has exposed chronic disparities in health, housing, and income throughout the county—issues that existed prior to the pandemic and have ultimately left Latinos more vulnerable to the virus.

Advocates and service providers who have long worked with Latinos say the pandemic's disproportionate impact on the population was inevitable, and in order to address Latino infection rates, the county and state not only needed to invest in outreach and expanded testing but provide solutions for some of the underlying issues that make Latinos more vulnerable, like job protections, financial and food assistance, and housing solutions.

"This all comes down to the inequities that existed, and this virus has exacerbated those," said Nancy Maldonado, CEO of the Chicano Federation. "It comes down to these structural inequities. What we're witnessing right now are the devastating consequences of not addressing them and not taking them seriously."

Kyra Greene, executive director of San Diego's Center for Policy Initiatives, said the most impacted ZIP codes in the county have both high concentrations of Latinos and poverty. Many of those ZIP codes are in South Bay.

"It's taken how extreme this disease is to highlight things that have always been challenges for some folks in our region," Greene said.

The Essential Workers

Many essential and high-contact job sectors are also staffed disproportionately by Latinos, meaning many work in jobs that may expose them more to the virus—positions they can't work remotely.

"A lot of these families are essential workers," said Maldonado. "So their risk increases and then the exposure to their entire families."

Latino employees are over-represented in grocery, convenience, and drug stores, childcare and social services, food service, and retail, according to SANDAG data.

Compared with the White population, Black and Latino populations are four times as likely to live in areas that have been hit hard by both COVID-19 and unemployment, SANDAG found in a June report. Compared with the Asian population, they are twice as likely to reside in areas with high COVID-19 cases and high unemployment.

Latinos also experienced higher poverty rates overall, compared with poverty rates countywide, prior to the pandemic. This makes them more likely to experience things like food insecurity and lower wages, which means if they have been exposed to COVID or experience mild symptoms, they are often faced with a decision between not going to work or being able to put food on their family's table.

"At the end of the day, they will choose to feed their families over their own health and safety," Maldonado said.

Maldonado said that for these families there need to be more wraparound services when someone tests positive.

"If someone is the sole bread winner in their family and tests positive, we need to have a support system in place, so they don't have to go to work," she said.

Abigail has been cleaning offices and hotels downtown for roughly 20 years. As the pandemic hit San Diego, she continued to go to work. She is a single mother and provides the sole income for her household. (Voice of San Diego is withholding Abigail's full name because of her immigration status.)

"My colleagues and I were living in fear that we would get sick," she said. "We were risking our health because we were essential workers."

In May, Abigail's fear turned into reality when she contracted COVID-19.

The struggle is particularly acute for unauthorized immigrant workers, like Abigail, who don't have access to any unemployment or other benefits.

Abigail said she is lucky. She had savings and union support, which provided her job protections and health insurance when she was sick.

In May, the state began distributing one-time payments of between $500 and $1,000 to some unauthorized immigrants. By June, Jewish Family Service had distributed $5 million to 10,000 people in the region, KPBS reported.

But the one-time payments haven't proven much for those who get sick or lose their jobs. Abigail did not receive state assistance.

"In reality, we have to continue to work to pay rent," Abigail said. "We're trying to make enough for food, to sustain our households. Some people have had their hours cut, are being paid less. But we get no help from the government."

Overcrowded Households

Latinos are also more likely than the county as a whole to live in crowded households.

During COVID times, that means when one person in a household gets sick, the disease can spread because family members can't isolate in a room.

Roughly 6.7 percent of people in San Diego County live in households with more than one person per room, according to 2018 census data. For Latinos in the county, that number increases to 17 percent.

One of the most impacted ZIP codes includes the San Ysidro Elementary School District, which has some of the highest rates of student homelessness in the county, a measure that includes families living in overcrowded or substandard conditions.

"It's difficult to have our parents quarantine and isolate if they have two families in an apartment," said Ana Melgoza, the vice president of external affairs at San Ysidro Health. "Just that alone is difficult."

Latino children are testing positive for the coronavirus at higher rates than other groups of children. Close contact with essential workers and crowded living conditions are to blame, CalMatters reported last month.

In situations where it is impossible to quarantine at home, people can call 211 or have their health care provider or community clinic help connect them to the county's public health hotel rooms, where they can isolate free of cost, said Barbara Jimenez, director of the central and southern regions for the county's Health and Human Services Agency.

But Melgoza said there hasn't been a good connection between the county's public health hotel room program and service providers on the front lines with these families, which has made moving individuals and families to those rooms difficult.

It's difficult to gauge how many Latino families are actually using the hotel rooms, though.

Of 1,272 people who have utilized the county public health hotel rooms 282 self-identified as Latino, according to data provided by the county. This data is largely incomplete, though, because the majority of occupants—736—did not report their ethnicity. The county also provided what language and translation request data was available, which showed 155 Spanish-speakers using the rooms.

Existing Health Disparities

Before the pandemic, Latinos already had relatively high rates of several health conditions like asthma, hypertension, diabetes, and heart disease that put them at greater risk of contracting COVID-19 and experiencing more severe symptoms.

Rates of diabetes and asthma were notably higher among Latinos compared with the county overall, according to a 2016 county report.

Rates of some communicable diseases, like the flu and pneumonia, were higher among Latinos than in the county overall, with Latinos in south county experiencing the highest rate among Latinos.

The same report also noted that in 2011, only 37 percent of Latino adults and children between six months and 11 years old said they had been vaccinated for the flu.

A 2014 county Community Health Assessment for the South Bay found that rates of diabetes death, hospitalization, and emergency department discharges in the region were higher among Latinos here than in other regions. Rates of heart disease deaths were also higher in communities of color in the southern parts of the county, the assessment found.

The county has been working to address the health disparities for years, said Jimenez.

"Many of these key issues are not new," Jimenez said. "These are areas that we have been working on, in particularly South County—rates of diabetes, obesity, unemployment factors, and housing factors."

The health realities not only put Latinos in the South Bay at risk of experiencing more dire outcomes with COVID-19, they could also create problems if people don't seek treatment for those conditions out of fear of the virus.

Ensuring that patients continue to get treatment for chronic conditions, like heart disease and hypertension, has been a priority for San Ysidro Health during the pandemic, said Dr. Maria Carriedo-Ceniceros, the organization's chief medical officer.

Carriedo-Ceniceros is also concerned about a wave of children who won't be vaccinated because their parents are fearful of coming to the doctor's office during the pandemic.

"Why we're more impacted by COVID-19 really goes back to the whole issue of existing health disparities in our community," Carriedo-Ceniceros said. "We serve a population that has high rates of diabetes, heart disease, hypertension. All of those have a high correlation with worse outcomes if a person contracts COVID."

Outreach Problems

Greene, the Center for Policy Initiatives executive director, divides the reasons as to why Latinos have been so highly impacted into two categories: challenges that existed pre-COVID that are exacerbated by the virus—like poverty and health issues—and challenges related to the way governments addressed COVID.

Advocates and service providers have noted a lack of outreach to the Latino community in the early stages of the pandemic to ensure they had information about the virus, how it could spread, and what assistance may be available to them. Greene said while outreach has significantly improved, it was lacking in the pandemic's early days.

The county could also have ramped up enforcement among employers earlier to help prevent the spread of the virus among essential workers, many of whom are Latino, Greene said. It wasn't always clear how a worker who felt pressure to show up to work could report that their working conditions were unsafe. Workers who walk off their job are not eligible for unemployment benefits.

The county only recently announced amped up enforcement efforts, like a call center where people can submit complaints.

"I'm glad to see the county step up," Maldonado said. "We just wish it would've happened sooner."

While Latinos make up 62 percent of COVID-19 cases, only 12.8 percent of county contact tracers—the workers who investigate where sick people have been and reach out to people who might have come into contact with them—and 14.6 percent of public health investigators speak Spanish, according to county data. The county data only reflects county employees and does not include roughly 100 additional contact tracers who have been hired as contractors.

Jimenez said a major focus of hers has been to get information out via radio, television, fliers, and word of mouth, through community leaders and promotores. She also said the county has been trying to make clear that in getting tested, accessing public health hotel rooms, and speaking with contact tracers that no one will be asked about their immigration status.

"As a Latina and someone who grew up in South Bay, the way me, my mother, and my neighbor receive information will all be different," Jimenez said. "The ongoing effort to share the resources and information is really important."

Kate Nucci
Black San Diegans Received a Quarter of All Coronavirus-Related Citations

This story was first published by Voice of San Diego.

July 13, 2020

The number of arrests and tickets in San Diego fell dramatically after the pandemic hit and public health officials ordered people to stay home. But not all groups were impacted equally by the enforcement of those rules.

A VOSD analysis of San Diego Police Department crime data shows that Black San Diegans were cited with nearly 24 percent of all coronavirus-related offenses, despite being 6.5 percent of the population. In other words, one of our every four violations of various emergency orders went to a Black person.

It wasn't just in the category of public health. At almost every level, from traffic violations to violent crime, Black San Diegans represented a disproportionately large share of the alleged offenders.

Khalid Alexander, founder of Pillars of the Community, a social justice organization, said he wasn't surprised to learn about the figures.

"That's reflective of the experience that I, and people who live in southeast San Diego, and honestly communities like southeast San Diego all over the world, have experienced," he said.

David Loy, legal director at the ACLU of San Diego and Imperial counties, also said the post-COVID arrest data was unconscionable but consistent with other data he's seen over the years. A previous VOSD analysis of police stop data from July 2018 to July 2019 revealed that Black drivers were more likely to be stopped than anyone else, but the searches resulted in lower or roughly the same rate of property seizures compared with other races. Those findings predated the pandemic and included both SDPD and the San Diego County Sheriff's Department.

Between January and March 12, the day before the county's shelter-in-place order went into effect, SDPD logged about 240 offenses on average every day, either through arrests or tickets. Between March 13 and May 30, they averaged 114 a day.

Arrests and tickets fell by half, and for nearly all categories of offenses. For example, between January and March 12, officers handed out 1,300 citations and arrests for loitering and trespassing. Between March 13 and May 30, that number dropped to 688.

Lieutenant Shawn Takeuchi, an SDPD spokesperson, said the city had made no changes to the way it goes about enforcing the laws on the books other than to require officers socially distance when possible and wear personal protective equipment. When asked why arrests and tickets have dropped by so much, he suggested I seek out a sociologist for comment.

Generally, the most common offense to spring up in the wake of the pandemic was a violation of the state emergency plan. The statute itself is fairly vague and Takeuchi did not respond to a follow-up request for clarification on what exactly it means to violate the state emergency orders.

Between January and June, Black San Diegans made up nearly 26 percent of all arrests and 14 percent of all citations.

After the pandemic hit, the data reveals especially great disparities in loitering and trespassing cases and disobeying a police officer. In both instances, Black San Diegans made up about 30 percent of all those cited.

While combing through the data, I spotted several other interesting trends.

Violent Crime Went Up

SDPD recorded 633 violent crimes before the pandemic and 707 after it began.

The number of domestic violence-related calls had dropped in February and March compared with the year before, but social workers expected it to rise as the pandemic wore on. And it appears that they were right.

The number of domestic violence-related reports rose slightly—especially offenses related to spousal abuse causing minor injury, which jumped from 121 to 199. General battery offenses, on the other hand, dropped from 105 cases reported to 69.

More Likely to Encounter Police, More Likely to Get Charged

I also separated out people whose names appeared four or more times in the data, oftentimes for offenses typically reserved for the homeless.

In total, 345 people were arrested or cited four or more times, making up 1,798 of the 25,634 offenses logged by SDPD from January to June. They received 992 collective citations before the pandemic's start and 806 after. Nearly 30 percent of all the repeat offenders were Black.

The most common offense for reported repeat violators, by far, was "unauthorized encroachment," which appeared 1,076 times. The law prohibits placing any personal objects on public sidewalks except for loading or unloading merchandise. It was meant to target errant trash dumpsters, but has been used instead to target the homeless.

The number of people cited specifically with unauthorized encroachment dropped from 664 to 412 after the start of the pandemic, a smaller drop than in other categories.

"Lodging without consent" was cited 550 times, making it the next most common. It dropped from 381 appearances pre-pandemic to 169 during it. Citations for violating vehicle habitation ordinances, meanwhile, dropped from 33 to 12.

Police said in April they are easing up on citations related to homelessness. A City Council resolution passed in early April also encouraged the mayor to impose a moratorium on charging people for sleeping in vehicles for the duration of the pandemic.

But SDPD and the mayor have defended their current level of enforcement against unsheltered people, arguing that their presence on the streets may also result in bad public health outcomes.

Jesse Marx

On the Eve of Being Back on His Feet, He Was Gone

This story was first published by Voice of San Diego.

January 6, 2022

Vincent Malijan came back to San Diego without much money or identification. It was the early months of the pandemic, and he had nowhere else to turn.

He'd recently suffered a stroke. Both his hand and his tongue were shaky, but he managed to place a phone call.

He was at a bus station and needed help.

None of Vincent's family members had room at the time—"we were all just barely getting by," said his sister-in-law Susan—so they found him a bed at the new homeless shelter inside the San Diego Convention Center. He could sleep there and work with a speech therapist while his relatives summoned bureaucratic alchemy to revive his livelihood on paper.

It helped that Susan had been a mail carrier downtown and already knew some of the service providers. But the family was unsure of where exactly to start, asking friends on social media for advice.

Getting Vincent back into the system was harder than it might sound. The process of re-establishing someone's official identity so they can get health care and other benefits has always been tedious. But it was compounded because of the pandemic and Vincent's physical condition.

He could barely talk or write, and his relatives didn't have the authority to advocate on his behalf. The shelter had to provide a waiver giving the family permission to share confidential information, which was part of the original calculus for placing him there.

Even then, the Malijans got the impression as they called around that officials were being bombarded with requests. At times they felt as though they were under suspicion—like they were trying to scam the government.

"To get him assistance was ridiculous," recalled Jeffrobert, his brother. "When I tried to explain to people on the phone, they would hang up on us."

After several months of pleading with administrators and filing forms, Vincent received medical treatment, Social Security, and other benefits. The whole process took six months.

As time rolled on, his relatives noticed an improvement in his mood and mobility. They bought him an electric bike and he started riding around town, beaming, they said, as he came up the hill toward their house.

"It was a blessing for him to reunite with the family," said Joseph, another brother. "Then he was taken away again."

By November, a room had become available in Joseph's home in Paradise Hills. But days before he was scheduled to move out of the Convention Center, Vincent tested positive for COVID-19. He spent the rest of his life in a hospital.

He died in late December without his loved ones by his side. The family took the little money Vincent had saved up and spent it on his cremation costs and a remembrance in his honor.

The excitement of the last few months turned to grief.

They feel today as though they were robbed. Being Vincent's caretaker brought them closer than ever. "We worked so hard during the time he was here," Jeffrobert said.

Vincent was one of at least 33 who succumbed to COVID and was later identified by the county as a person experiencing homelessness. The term "homeless" is fluid. Someone, for instance, may have been couch surfing when they got sick.

But several of the death certificates Voice of San Diego reviewed as part of its examination of the first year of the pandemic clearly identify the person's living status. Some list an intersection downtown as the last-known address. Another simply states: "unsheltered streets of San Diego."

Early in the pandemic, case rates among homeless residents were lower than expected. Observers credited the city's decision to move people out of shelters and into the Convention Center. Some also ended up in hotel rooms to mitigate the risk of spreading the virus to others.

Officials said they'd learned from the deadly hepatitis A outbreak only a few years prior and continued to keep the Convention Center open despite calls from advocates and public health experts—around the same time Vincent was in the hospital—to move more people into individual spaces. Critics argued that putting hundreds of vulnerable folks in a single place was a ticking time bomb.

By 2021, the Regional Task Force on Homelessness reported that the hospitalization rate for people experiencing homelessness was much higher than the general population. An outbreak, some said, was inevitable, but by quickly turning the Convention Center into a shelter officials had protected and ultimately saved lives.

Still, as well-intentioned as the region's response may have been, there were larger forces at play that made living without stable housing more fraught and precarious than ever before.

The homeless people who contracted the coronavirus were more likely to perish at a younger age. County data show that the median age of someone who died of COVID since the start of the pandemic was 76.

But when homeless people are separated from the wider population, the median age of death drops to 62.

The gap is startling but mirrors what we already know about the extreme toll that homelessness can take on the human mind and body.

The major causes of death for homeless people under 45 tend to be related to substance abuse, mental health, and assault. Those who make it into their 50s and beyond tend to die from the same conditions that plague the wider population, but decades sooner.

Dr. Margot Kushel, a physician at UC San Francisco who studies vulnerable communities, has found that homeless people age at a much quicker rate. Many grew up poor and accumulated a lifetime of toxic stress. They typically suffer from poor nutrition and a lack of access to health care. Some served time in jail. Some worked physically demanding jobs earlier in life.

"Homeless people in their 50s, they really look in every measure like people who are in their 70s," Kushel told me. "Homeless people in their 60s look more like people in their 80s."

Vincent was 69 when he passed. He had been born in Guam and raised in National City in a big family. Relatives described Vincent's father as an austere man, a dishwasher in the Navy who didn't make much money and who would physically punish his children.

Vincent started a family of his own, got divorced, and ended up in Long Beach in the 1990s working jobs in the shipyards and elsewhere. That's when his life really fell apart. He was arrested and sentenced as part of a drug trafficking case.

Prosecutors alleged that James Cabaccang and his two brothers had transported large quantities of methamphetamine from California to Guam. The defendants maintained for years that they had been railroaded, and the Ninth Circuit Court of Appeals ended up reversing part of the conviction.

The federal government netted $500,000 after seizing jewels, cars, and money, one newspaper reported. James Cabaccang got life in prison for what appear to be non-violent offenses. Two decades later, President Barack Obama commuted Cabaccang's sentence as one of his last acts in office.

At trial, one of the Cabaccang brothers had been accused of recruiting people to fly from Los Angeles to Guam with packages of methamphetamine under their clothing, then wire the money back.

Vincent's role in the conspiracy is murky because the court records are sealed. The family members I spoke to said they didn't know the details of the case, only that Vincent had gotten himself involved in something bad. He was one of at least nine defendants and tight with the Cabaccangs.

Vincent's son, Christopher, was a teenager at the time and remembered how he used to sit on a stool in the bar that the family ran. The feds took the bar too, he said.

Vincent got 15 years behind bars and was shipped to Arizona in 2010 to serve out his probation. He did another brief stint in jail for failing to tell his probation officer about a change of address. After that, he was booted back into civil society—a free man, at least in theory. The conviction made it difficult to find housing or a job. He didn't have any specific skills he could lean on and by then he was in his late 50s.

"It fucked up his life," Christopher said. "With his record, who would hire him? He hid it because he was ashamed."

The two stayed in touch as Vincent moved around the Southwest. For a time, he landed in a trailer park, but his girlfriend, according to multiple family members, died before the pandemic hit.

In June 2020, Vincent took a one-way trip to San Diego.

Despite the awful circumstances, Vincent's return gave his family the chance to squash any lingering tension. Christopher, in particular, had plenty of pent-up resentment toward his father, but he took care of him and loved him nonetheless.

"I could see his remorse, his grief, his sorrow," Christopher said. "It was just the way he looked at me. He would cry and get real emotional, like, 'I wish I could have done more for you.'"

I spoke to Christopher on the one-year anniversary of his father's death. The day before, he and others had held a barbecue in Vincent's memory, so they could say goodbye and repeat some of the old jokes they'd told about the old man over the years—how he'd shake your hand and steal your wallet.

Rather than a mourning, the gathering was a celebration of a rough-and-tumble life, warts and all. Christopher took to Facebook that same day for some healthy shit-talking. "Never Forget," he posted alongside a photograph of Vincent wearing tie-dye. "Dad, brother, uncle, friend, menace, u get the point."

He certainly made an impression on the staff at the shelter. Bob McElroy, CEO of Alpha Project, said Vincent was a sweet guy and well-liked. It helped that his family cared enough about him to serve as his translator when others couldn't understand him.

By all accounts, Vincent was highly motivated to get better. And just like that, on the eve of being back on his own feet, he was gone—something that happens with alarming regularity, even if the general public is oblivious of its own underbelly and the effort it takes to pull people out of destitution.

"I see it every day," McElroy said. "You could take that story and add a hundred to it."

Maya Srikrishnan
Local Vaccine Rates Highlight Barriers Facing Black and Latino Communities

This story was first published by Voice of San Diego.

February 19, 2021

Bertha Garcia has been trying to get an appointment for her COVID-19 vaccine for about a month.

Garcia, who qualifies for the vaccine because of her community work with the Chicano Foundation, said she tried day after day to get an appointment, but couldn't.

"I tried different dates," she said. "I tried to do the same date again. They always ask me for my information, but once I put it in, it will say there aren't any more appointments."

Garcia had heard some people had luck trying to make appointments in the middle of the night, but waking up at midnight just isn't an option for her.

"I'm going to continue to try," she said. "The most frustrating thing to me is that I have experience with a computer. I can't imagine people who don't have that experience, don't have anyone to help, and keep filling this out, to be told they can't make an appointment."

Getting an appointment is one of the biggest—but not the only—obstacle that many in marginalized communities have been facing as they try to obtain the coronavirus vaccine.

Although Latinos currently make up 56 percent of coronavirus cases—and in the past have made up even higher percentages of cases—

and nearly 44 percent of deaths in the county, more than any other racial or ethnic group, they represent just over 15 percent of vaccinations, according to county data. Only 2 percent of vaccines have gone to Black people, while they make up 5 percent of the county's population. Latinos and Blacks have the lowest vaccination rates in the county. Only 61.7 people per every 1,000 Black people are being vaccinated, and 73.5 per every 1,000 Latinos are being vaccinated. For White people, that number is 154.6 per 1,000 people and for Asians, it is 131.7 per 1,000.

County spokeswoman Sarah Sweeney noted that the county is tied to the state's tier system for vaccine distribution, which limits who is eligible for the vaccine. Sweeney also said that more than a quarter of people vaccinated declined to provide race or ethnicity data to the county or selected "mixed race."

Community organizations say the discrepancy is fueled by access and trust issues that Latinos and Blacks face. The technological savviness and time needed to get a vaccine appointment is one barrier. Issues with language access or transportation are others. There's also distrust—between Black people in the U.S. and medicine—and residual fear from the Trump administration for Latinos.

"We just went through this with testing," said Nancy Maldonado, CEO of the Chicano Foundation. "It feels like we've learned nothing."

Barriers to Access Are Higher for Latinos and Blacks

Tere Olivas had been trying for two weeks to get a vaccine appointment for her husband, who is 73. Olivas and her husband live in the 92114 ZIP code or the Skyline area, which has had one of the highest COVID rates in the county.

Olivas and her husband have been in a strict lockdown since last March, she said. At 63 years old, she still doesn't qualify for a vaccine, but once her husband was eligible, she made an effort to get him an appointment. There were roughly a dozen locations they could have gone to, but she couldn't get an appointment at any of them.

"I would try at 8 at night, at noon, at 10 in the morning," Olivas said in Spanish. "I kept getting no. There are no appointments, there are no appointments."

Finally on Wednesday, Olivas and her husband decided to try their luck by simply showing up to a site.

They got lucky.

Although Olivas didn't have an appointment, volunteers at the vaccination station in Chula Vista were able to help them make one on the spot. Her husband was vaccinated within an hour.

This week, Sharp Health-run vaccine sites opened up 2,000 appointments—a boon for many like Garcia and Olivas who had been struggling to make an appointment.

"The majority of people who have gotten vaccines are White," said Dr. Rodney Hood, a physician and president of the Multicultural Health Foundation. "It's open to everyone who is knowledgeable and can get on their phone. It's a race."

The county rolled out a program this week that will set aside appointments at vaccination sites in Chula Vista, San Ysidro, National City, and Imperial Beach for community groups who have community health workers, or promotoras, working with at-risk communities that have historically had difficulties accessing resources during the pandemic.

"Recognizing the historic inequities in vulnerable populations, outreach and promotion efforts include utilizing the county's existing network of promotoras and community health workers who have shared backgrounds and experiences with the diverse population in San Diego," Sweeney, the county spokeswoman, wrote in an email. "Their efforts include, among a wide variety of other things, assisting individuals in scheduling vaccination appointments."

That's a start, Maldonado said. Her staff had been trying to assist community members in scheduling appointments and had run into availability issues.

While there have been improvements in accessing appointments, Maldonado said that the weeks missed have an impact, just like they did when testing was rolled out later in certain communities at the beginning of the pandemic.

There are multiple factors that have made vaccine access particularly elusive for elder Latinos, she said.

"One is computer literacy and being computer-savvy," Maldonado said. "But also having to sit at the computer and hit refresh repeatedly or wait on hold for hours with 211. If you think about Latino families, most of the younger generations are working still, so it's not like they have people who can spend hours with them helping to get their appointment."

Transportation presents another barrier even once someone has secured an appointment. Some of the vaccine locations are accessible by public transit, but that doesn't mean getting there is easy or quick. Plus, some elderly people may be fearful of taking public transportation right now. Many younger generations in Black and Latino communities are essential workers, so there are limited timeframes during which they can give their elder family members a ride.

The highest concentration of vaccination sites is near and around South County, Sweeney said. There are vaccination sites in Imperial Beach, San Ysidro, Chula Vista, National City, and Southeastern San Diego. A site in Lemon Grove will also be coming online on February 21, she said.

The largest percentage of vaccines—21.7 percent—have been distributed in the county's North Central region, which includes areas like La Jolla, Scripps Ranch, Pacific Beach, and Point Loma. The South region, which includes hard-hit areas like Chula Vista, National City, Otay

Mesa, and San Ysidro, makes up 15.1 percent of the total vaccines distributed so far, according to county data.

That's an improvement, said Hood, "but we still think it is a problem."

Both the Multicultural Health Foundation and Chicano Federation are working with the county to reach vulnerable communities but say there still aren't enough community health workers to truly ensure everyone eligible for a vaccine in those communities has access to it.

The Chicano Federation is getting up to 100 calls some days seeking help scheduling vaccine appointments.

Maldonado also warned that the county should be thinking of how to administer second doses of the vaccine to these communities.

"There will be challenges that come up with making sure people get that second dose," she said. "We're already seeing appointments starting to come up for second doses, but most of those come through email, so if you don't check your email or don't have an email address, you won't see it. We need to think that far ahead to make sure those people don't just get missed completely and that there is some sort of follow-up."

The Importance of Trust and Information

A long history of abuse and neglect in the U.S. medical system is also keeping some Black people from even wanting the vaccine if they are eligible, Hood said.

According to a countywide survey conducted in December and January by FM3 Research about vaccine attitudes, 36 percent of African-Americans said they were unlikely to take the vaccine. That's higher than any other race.

"Black issues especially go back to centuries of inhumane treatment in America. People often mention Tuskegee, but that's just the tip of the iceberg," said Hood, referring to a public health study in which Black men were injected with syphilis without their knowledge or consent.

In the Latino community, Maldonado said, community health workers have had to dispel misinformation and rumors that can spread quickly.

"People were hearing that there were really intense side effects," Maldonado said. "There were rumors that there were quite a few number of deaths related to the vaccine. A few people had heard it had affected women's ability to get pregnant. Those kinds of things were already circulated before we really started talking about the vaccine as community health workers. It got way ahead of us."

Fatima Muñoz, director of research and health promotion for San Ysidro Health, said she's heard many questions about whether the vaccine is safe and why it was developed so quickly.

"It's really important that the community can get information from organizations and people that they trust," Muñoz said.

Both Muñoz and Maldonado said that they've seen people's attitudes toward the vaccine change with increased education about it. Hood also emphasized the importance of trusted messengers within the Black community to educate people about the vaccine.

But trust issues go beyond just information about the vaccine.

One issue that may be deterring immigrants in the community from accessing the vaccine is the fact that some websites ask for people's Social Security numbers when they try to sign up for an appointment. It's not actually necessary to provide a Social Security number—you can just enter all zeros—but the question itself raises a red flag for many who fear interactions with the government could trigger immigration enforcement, said Muñoz and Maldonado.

"People don't know that it isn't mandatory, so when they see it, it's a barrier," Muñoz said.

Lingering fear and distrust Latino immigrants feel from the Trump administration is also playing into efforts to distribute vaccines to the community.

"People want to know who this information is going to be shared with, and will it be obvious if they put in all zeros that they don't have a Social Security number? I know that's been a deterrent," Maldonado said.

Although the Department of Homeland Security has indicated it will not be patrolling or monitoring vaccine sites, many Latino immigrants are still nervous about going to them.

"We're heard many people say, 'We want to wait until somewhere smaller in my neighborhood opens up,'" Maldonado said.

Indeed, the county vaccine attitude survey also indicated that residents of all races and ethnicities are most comfortable getting the vaccine at their doctor's office, followed by a pharmacy or a medical clinic in their community. Only 25 percent of survey respondents said they would feel comfortable going to a pop-up vaccination clinic or a library or community center.

"It's great to have a superstation, but how can we engage our community enough that they will go through the door and get the vaccine?" Muñoz said.

As the county works to increase vaccination sites, Muñoz says it's critical that community organizations like hers continue to build trust and provide information.

"Every time there is a challenge, we need to recognize it and inform our community," she said. "Things are getting better—and I'm glad—but we have to do better as a county to really ensure that we can improve trust with our community. It's not only providing the resources, but also providing the appropriate information in the way our community deserves to get it."

prison

Jill Castellano and Mary Plummer
County Jail Workers Prioritized for Vaccines While Inmates Have to Wait

> *This story was originally produced and published by inewsource, a nonprofit, nonpartisan newsroom in San Diego committed to exposing wrongdoing and holding powerful people and institutions accountable. As part of their commitment to keeping the San Diego community informed, inewsource has allowed this story to be reprinted and shared here with you. To learn more about their work and how you can support their journalism, visit inewsource.org.*

March 13, 2021

San Diego County has prioritized corrections officers for COVID-19 vaccines while thousands of inmates haven't been offered doses.

About 4,000 people are locked in one of the county's seven jails each day, and because of high turnover and short sentences, many more come into contact with these detention centers each month. Yet only 26 inmates have been inoculated since January, according to data the Sheriff's Department provided Wednesday.

The low vaccination rates could signal trouble. Because people cycle in and out of jails quickly, inmates are potential vectors who can carry the virus from detention centers into neighborhoods. Research has linked jails and prisons to high infection rates in nearby communities.

More than 1,200 people in San Diego County jails have tested positive for COVID-19 since the pandemic began.

The vaccinated inmates include five people who were discharged after getting their first dose and 10 still incarcerated who have yet to receive their second dose.

Meanwhile, 476 jail workers have received at least one shot from the sheriff's medical services division, according to the data. That adds up to roughly a quarter of corrections employees.

Staff who were vaccinated through other means aren't included in the numbers—nor are those who participated in a "zero-waste" vaccine program offered by Cal Fire San Diego, which was giving spare doses to law enforcement officers before they were eligible.

"It's really devastating, actually, to hear that so few people in jail have been vaccinated," said Naomi Sugie, an associate criminology professor at UC Irvine.

"It is really good that the employees are getting vaccinated at such high rates, but we have to give the same sort of priority, out of public health concerns, to people who are incarcerated in those facilities," Sugie said.

The county public health department opened vaccinations to law enforcement officers on February 27, but only inmates who are 65 and older were eligible. Lieutenant Ricardo Lopez, a Sheriff's Department spokesperson, said everyone in that age group has been offered vaccines, and 25 declined.

Lopez said the department follows county and state guidelines and offers inmates vaccines as soon as they're available.

"It's all depending on when we get the vaccines from the county," he said.

While hundreds of corrections staff received vaccines in February and March, an outbreak was spreading at George Bailey Detention Facility in Otay Mesa. A man booked in mid-February for driving under the influence was transferred to the jail and began showing COVID-19 symptoms, according to the Sheriff's Department. At least 47 inmates have tested positive for the virus since then.

The county is following state guidelines, which were updated this week to include all inmates in the next phase of vaccinations that starts on Monday, spokesperson Sarah Sweeney said.

This is happening as the county continues to struggle to secure enough doses for those who are already on the priority list. A shortage of vaccines has forced local officials to repeatedly close public vaccination sites and prioritize those who haven't been able to get their second shots.

To prevent outbreaks, some counties have jumped ahead of the state's plan and already offered vaccinations to all of their inmates. Sacramento, Santa Clara and Contra Costa counties have done so, but San Diego County has not. Its vaccine rollout plan doesn't mention jails.

"There's really no reason to be prioritizing corrections staff over people who have these vulnerabilities, who are inside jails and prisons," said Wanda Bertram, a spokesperson at the national nonprofit Prison Policy Initiative.

Federal agencies acknowledge people in detention centers have higher rates of many medical conditions, which make them more susceptible to COVID-19. And because they live in confined quarters, the virus can spread easily once inside the facilities.

More than 1,200 people in San Diego County jails have tested positive for COVID-19 since the pandemic began, and the Sheriff's Department has acknowledged one inmate death from the virus. At least 553 department employees, including those who don't work in the jails, have contracted it, and one has died.

In a class-action lawsuit filed this week, the San Diego chapter of the American Civil Liberties Union claimed Sheriff Bill Gore and his department have inflicted cruel and unusual punishment on inmates by housing them in crowded, unsanitary spaces without adequate medical care. It demands inmates receive vaccines as soon as possible and jail populations be reduced to prevent the spread of the virus.

"There is no reasonable dispute about the importance of vaccines and the urgent need for prompt vaccination," the lawsuit says.

The ACLU co-filed the suit with a San Diego law firm and a social justice advocacy group co-founded by Geneviéve Jones-Wright, a former deputy public defender who ran for county district attorney in 2018.

Their complaint tells the story of Terry Leroy Jones, who lives in the medical housing unit of the George Bailey Detention Facility because of his asthma, diabetes, and prosthetic leg. The 55-year-old is jailed on a home invasion robbery charge.

A man with COVID-19 symptoms was placed in Jones's unit for three days before testing positive, the lawsuit says, causing him and most of the other inmates in nearby bunks to catch the virus.

Jones "would like vaccines to be made available to people incarcerated in the jails to help prevent COVID-19 from continuing to spread, especially because of how frequently people are moved around the facilities," according to the lawsuit. "But jail staff have never said anything about the vaccines to him, and he knows about them only because of the news."

The suit also says corrections staff have told inmates "they will be the last in line to receive a vaccine."

At California prisons, more than 42,000 inmates and 25,000 staff have been vaccinated. A spokesperson for the Richard J. Donovan Correctional Facility deferred questions to the state agency that handles healthcare in prisons, which refused to say how many inmates at the prison in Otay Mesa have received vaccines.

The facility has seen nearly 1,000 infections, and the state's COVID-19 tracker shows 18 deaths.

"We know how horrible these conditions are, and yet we subject people to them without batting an eye," said Khalid Alexander, president and founder of Pillars of the Community, a San Diego nonprofit advocating for change in the criminal justice system.

"If you take away someone's ability to stay healthy," he said, "if you take away someone's ability to do any kind of the basic care for their basic needs, whose responsibility is it?"

Sofía Mejías-Pascoe
COVID-19 Cases at San Diego's ICE Detention Center Reach All-Time High

> *This story was originally produced and published by inewsource, a nonprofit, nonpartisan newsroom in San Diego committed to exposing wrongdoing and holding powerful people and institutions accountable. As part of their commitment to keeping the San Diego community informed, inewsource has allowed this story to be reprinted and shared here with you. To learn more about their work and how you can support their journalism, visit inewsource.org.*

January 18, 2022

A San Diego detention center that houses U.S. Immigration and Customs Enforcement detainees saw COVID-19 cases surge last week, reporting the third highest number of active cases among ICE detainees at any of the federal agency's more than 130 detention centers.

On January 10, the Otay Mesa Detention Center reported having 91 people in isolation or being monitored with confirmed cases, ICE reported in online data. That number was an all-time high for the San Diego facility and was surpassed only by facilities in Arizona and Texas, similarly situated near the U.S.–Mexico border.

The infections account for about 10% of ICE detainees at the facility based on population numbers that an attorney with the American Civil Liberties Union of San Diego and Imperial Counties said the agency provided at the beginning of this month.

The ACLU receives data regularly from the ICE facility, located in southern San Diego County just three miles from the U.S.–Mexico border, as part of an agreement in a lawsuit over COVID-19 protections at the facility.

The case counts fluctuate daily. The 91 reported active cases among detainees as of January 10 fell to 52 by Sunday, according to ICE's website.

However, the outbreak still represents the highest active case count among ICE detainees in the facility since the pandemic began, according to case counts tracked by UCLA. It comes amid a recent increase in immigrant arrivals at the southern border while cases of the omicron variant skyrocket across the United States. It is one of several ICE facilities situated along the U.S.–Mexico border that is experiencing high case counts.

An attorney for the ACLU said there are more than 500 medically vulnerable detainees housed at Otay Mesa, whose population has doubled in less than a year. Many of those detainees could be released under an existing court order, he said.

A lack of clear data around who is tested and vaccinated within the facilities raises questions about how protected detainees are from the outbreak, experts said.

"We're concerned about the health and safety of the people inside, and we're concerned about the health and safety of people in the surrounding communities," said Joshua Manson, communications manager for UCLA School of Law's COVID Behind Bars Data Project.

"We know that outbreaks don't stay behind prison or detention center walls."

The border facility, which houses migrants awaiting court dates or deportation and federal inmates under U.S. Marshals Service custody awaiting trials or sentencing, is owned and operated by CoreCivic, a private detention and corrections management company that operates six facilities in California and more than 100 across the United States.

There are 17 active cases among its employees at Otay Mesa as of January 12, according to data posted on the company's website.

A spokesperson for ICE declined to comment on questions from inewsource about the outbreak but said the agency "remains committed to applying CDC guidance and providing vaccine education that ensures those in our care and custody can make an informed choice during this global pandemic."

The U.S. Marshals Service did not answer specific questions about the outbreak but said through a spokesperson that facilities that house federal inmates, including the Otay Mesa Detention Center, "are responsible for the medical care that prisoners receive."

"All training protocols, quarantine decisions, or policy adjustments are made at the facility level," Lynzey Donahue, spokesperson for the U.S. Marshals said in an email.

COVID-19 Cases Surge

While active cases started to decline at Otay Mesa toward the end of last week, the outbreak represents the facility's largest since the pandemic began and comes while its detainee population is more than twice what it was less than a year ago.

More than 750 people have tested positive for COVID-19 while at the facility, as of January 17. One ICE detainee died from the virus in May 2020.

At the end of December, ICE reported six COVID-19 cases among the facility's detainees. By the next week, that number was up to 36.

Less than a week after that, the agency reported 91 active cases among detainees—the highest active case count yet, according to the UCLA School of Law's COVID Behind Bars Data Project, which has collected data reported by corrections and detention agencies over the course of the pandemic.

The facility's previous outbreaks were less than half the size of the most recent one. The second highest active case count at the facility was reported in July 2021 with 44 cases, according to UCLA data.

Ryan Gustin, a spokesperson for CoreCivic, said "many of the current active cases" at Otay Mesa include migrants who entered the facility already infected with the virus.

"With the recent increase of immigrants entering the United States along our southern border, we have seen a similar increase in the number of detainees that are arriving to our facilities already positive for COVID-19," Gustin said in an email.

Border Patrol encounters in the San Diego sector in October were double what they were the year before, according to the latest available online data.

Monthly encounters increased from September to October by 13%, then decreased the following month by 6% for a total of 13,416 encounters in November 2021.

But quarantines resulting from the latest outbreak have affected long-term detainees as well.

Lilia Rodriguez, an immigration attorney in San Diego, said her client, a 34-year-old man from Nicaragua who's been detained at Otay Mesa for nearly six months, was forced to miss a special bond hearing that could have allowed him to be released from detention at the facility.

Rodriguez said not all housing units have the equipment needed to attend court appearances or meet with attorneys virtually. That means court proceedings are often delayed for those quarantined in units without the equipment.

"It does really, really hinder how they can find ways to get out of detention and proceed with their cases, so it's just frustrating for them and for us," Rodriguez said.

Rodriguez said the quarantines can also be extended multiple times, further delaying her clients' proceedings.

CoreCivic did not answer specific questions about how many housing units or detainees at the facility are currently under quarantine. CoreCivic and ICE officials said the facility tests new detainees and inmates upon arrival and houses them separately from the general population for two weeks.

The number of ICE detainees at Otay Mesa has fluctuated over the course of the pandemic but is now up to 810 as of early January, according to data from the ACLU. Nearly a year prior, in February 2021, that number was down to 332.

ICE declined to provide information about the number of detainees currently at the facility due to "security concerns." However, ICE provides population numbers and other data regularly to the ACLU as part of an agreement in a class action lawsuit over COVID-19 protections at the facility and the Imperial Regional Detention Facility.

It's concerning to Bardis Vakili, senior staff attorney at the ACLU of San Diego and Imperial Counties, that the detainee population size has swelled as much as it has, particularly because more than two-thirds of that population are medically vulnerable.

In the pandemic's first year, a U.S. District Court judge ordered ICE to identify and consider releasing detainees who were medically vulnerable to COVID-19. That order is ongoing and applies to ICE facilities across the country.

Now, though, Vakili said there are about 540 medically vulnerable detainees at Otay Mesa who meet the standards set in that case, Fraihat, et al. v. U.S. Immigration and Customs Enforcement, that have not been released yet.

"That's a lot of risk you're imposing on several hundred people who are at the mercy of the people who are taking them into custody," Vakili said.

That number comes from the data reports the ACLU receives from the facility. CoreCivic's medical staff confirms the conditions that make detainees vulnerable to COVID-19 as they arrive at the facility or while they are detained.

ICE did not answer questions about those detainees or why they had not been released.

Manson, with the UCLA COVID Behind Bars Data Project, said that after two years of collecting data on COVID-19 testing and cases at federal, state, and local incarceration facilities, he sees the way to prevent large outbreaks.

"The best measure that can be taken to address COVID-19 in congregate settings, including in prisons and detention centers, is decarceration and decreasing population density," Manson said.

Vaccination and the Risk of Community Spread

Murky information about vaccinations among ICE detainees raises questions about who is protected from the virus.

ICE's national vaccination campaign was criticized for being inconsistent across facilities and not providing a clear picture of vaccination rates and accessibility for detainees.

A report published in September from Homeland Security's inspector general found that Otay Mesa complied with standards for classifying detainee risk levels and provided adequate medical care. However, it also found that the facility "compromised the health, safety, and rights of detainees" by failing to enforce COVID-19 precautions like mask-wearing and social distancing.

In response, a top ICE official reported that medical staff at Otay Mesa had administered more than 750 doses of the vaccines to detainees by mid-August.

ICE has since then declined to provide inewsource with an updated number of vaccine administrations at Otay Mesa. A spokesperson for the agency said across its facilities, "48,246 noncitizens elected to receive

COVID-19 vaccinations" as of January 5. The agency said it began providing detainees with booster shots in November.

Vakili, the ACLU attorney, said there's been some confusion among detainees about vaccinations. He said some have called his team asking basic questions about boosters and the types of vaccines offered.

"This is a population that may not have a lot of access to information prior to getting there. And so it's really important to educate folks about vaccines so they can make informed health decisions," Vakili said.

Manson shares those concerns.

"It's not clear that people in its custody are being given proper educational materials and information in the right language about the vaccination, and we think that that's really paramount for the health and safety of people inside the facilities and in surrounding communities."

Gustin said CoreCivic detainees are provided information about vaccines during intake and with digital tablets that have information in more than a dozen languages. The company said it has held numerous vaccination events where detainees and employees can get vaccinated.

All of the company's employees at Otay Mesa are either partially or fully vaccinated, Gustin said.

The agency does not post vaccinations rates for its facilities publicly, and turnover among detainees at Otay Mesa complicates getting a clear picture of how much of the population is vaccinated at any point in time.

In the 2021 fiscal year, the average length of stay in ICE custody was 37 days, according to the agency. But while some detainees are there for months, others filter in and out of the facility in a matter of days, keeping the average length of stay low, said Vakili, the ACLU attorney.

"We have been in contact with people that have been there for the entirety of the pandemic," Vakili said. "The need to vaccinate them, the need to ensure they have access to boosters to continue to protect them, is really critical."

Jill Castellano and Mary Plummer
Donovan Deaths: 3 Prisoners Found Dead or Dying in Cells From COVID-19

> *This story was originally produced and published by inewsource, a nonprofit, nonpartisan newsroom in San Diego committed to exposing wrongdoing and holding powerful people and institutions accountable. As part of their commitment to keeping the San Diego community informed, inewsource has allowed this story to be reprinted and shared here with you. To learn more about their work and how you can support their journalism, visit inewsource.org.*

April 8, 2021

The crisis peaked four days before Christmas. San Diego's only prison was teeming with COVID-19 infections. A fifth of the 3,500 people incarcerated were sick, and many were relocated to three large gymnasiums so staff could reach them quickly in an emergency.

Over the next five weeks, 18 inmates died from the virus.

Through county medical examiner reports, death certificates and interviews, inewsource pieced together how these people lost their lives to COVID-19 while under the care of the Richard J. Donovan Correctional Facility in Otay Mesa.

Three of the inmates were found unresponsive in their cells, inewsource has learned, despite the corrections department insisting that those with COVID-19 are regularly monitored and transferred to hospitals if they need more intense care.

The cellmate of one of the men who died, Gilbert Rodriguez, said the 66-year-old was denied medical treatment from prison staff after testing positive and coughing through the night. Prison officials refused to respond to specific questions about his December 26 death.

"There is no crime that heinous that it sentences you to die of a virus and to not get medical attention," said Hadar Aviram, a criminologist and professor at the UC Hastings College of Law in San Francisco.

Court filings indicate Donovan has among the worst track records of California's 35 adult prisons in its response to the pandemic. The facility has acknowledged housing COVID-positive inmates with people who didn't have the virus because the staff was overwhelmed by the winter outbreak. It was also the only prison out of compliance with court orders to create enough wheelchair accessible beds in COVID-19 isolation areas when the surge in cases began.

The state's prison oversight office found Donovan had issued its staff the most written citations in December of any prison for refusing to wear masks or practice social distancing. The prison is now tied for the third-most coronavirus deaths in the state.

The California Department of Corrections and Rehabilitation wouldn't answer questions about individuals' healthcare or deaths, citing medical privacy concerns. Marcus Pollard, the warden at Donovan prison, declined multiple interview requests through a spokesperson. The department only responded to questions from inewsource over email.

"We have worked tirelessly to implement measures in the face of a brand-new virus and the inherent constraints that exist with a critical 24/7 operation," said Terri Hardy, a spokesperson for the state prison system.

Eight Days

The three men found in their cells, all 65 or older with pre-existing medical conditions, died within eight days of each other. Five other Donovan prisoners died at hospitals during that time.

Donovan guards discovered Ronald Johnson unresponsive in his single cell on the night of January 2. San Diego County medical examiner reports show he had recently been diagnosed with COVID-19.

Johnson was moved to a triage room as the guards attempted CPR and called 911. When the paramedics arrived, they couldn't save him.

"Nobody should be dying alone in a cell," said Rebecca Fielding-Miller, an assistant professor of public health at UC San Diego, after learning about inewsource's findings.

"There's a lot of things you can do to prevent that," she added.

Fielding-Miller said prisons should use frequent monitoring and testing to identify those who need more serious medical care. Plus, reducing the number of people incarcerated has proven to be an effective prevention tool that has not been fully used, she said.

Statewide, thousands of incarcerated people have been released from California prisons ahead of schedule, but advocates have called on officials to do more. In October, a state appeals court demanded San Quentin State Prison in Marin County cut its population in half after more than 2,000 inmates became sick.

A corrections department spokesperson said prisoners with COVID-19 are screened twice a day by medical staff. But its healthcare guidelines say infected inmates may need more attention than that because their conditions can deteriorate quickly—especially for those with underlying conditions who are showing symptoms.

When Johnson died, he was 69 and had lung disease, hypertension, and cirrhosis, medical examiner records show. The Vietnam War veteran also suffered from PTSD, paranoia, bipolar disorder, and narcotics addiction, according to a transcript from his 2016 parole board hearing. He needed a walker to help with his mobility.

Johnson was incarcerated for a 1992 drunken driving crash that killed four people in Fontana. He was scheduled for another parole hearing in

February, less than two months after he died from COVID-19 inside the prison.

"This punishment is not in the California penal code," Aviram said. "Not even for people that are sentenced to death. This is not fair. This is not the way to treat other human beings."

Aviram said prison medical staff across the state have struggled to keep up with the number of COVID-19 infections, making it possible for their seriously ill patients' conditions to worsen unattended.

"The kind of healthcare that you get in prison, it's not really healthcare," she said.

Gravely Ill

Ryan Rodriguez was shocked when he got the news the day after Christmas from his brother, who said the prison had called to inform them of their father's death. Rodriguez had spoken with his father about a week earlier.

Gilbert Rodriguez tested positive for COVID-19 at Donovan on December 23, medical examiner records show. He died three days later.

The family asked for details about Gilbert's condition in the days leading up to his death, but the prison wouldn't elaborate.

"Was he ever seen by a doctor?" Ryan Rodriguez said. "Was he ever put on any kind of ventilation? Was he ever put on any kind of meds? None of those answers were given to us."

About a month later, he received a letter from his father's cellmate, which said Gilbert had been coughing a lot after his diagnosis, and when he asked for medicine to soothe his throat, the staff did not give him any.

The coughing continued, the cellmate's letter says, and Gilbert got almost no sleep two nights in a row. Then, he experienced what looked like symptoms of a heart attack or stroke, according to the letter, and died.

His dying wish was for his two sons to know about the lack of medical help available inside the prison, the letter says.

"I would expect anybody with underlying conditions getting COVID [to] be monitored and tracked at some level, not just left in a cell and say, 'Good luck,'" Ryan Rodriguez said.

In March, Gilbert's son received an email from the Medical Examiner's Office with some of the only details he's been told about his father's illness. Healthcare staff made rounds and checked his father's vitals every day, it said.

Medical records show Gilbert had diabetes and cardiovascular disease. He was also an addict who struggled at times with drugs and alcohol, his son said.

He was serving a life sentence with the possibility of parole for lewd and lascivious acts conducted with a child under 14.

People in prison are mostly there for a reason, his son said.

"I don't expect them to be treated with white gloves, but I do feel like there should be something in place to address the situation when people become gravely ill," Ryan Rodriguez said.

Susceptible to Spread

Experts have noticed a troubling trend in California prisons—incarcerated people are refusing testing out of concerns they will be forced into isolation areas, which can be highly restrictive and similar to solitary confinement settings.

Penny Godbold, a San Francisco attorney who represents incarcerated people with disabilities, said her clients across the state have feared being transferred into isolation areas that don't accommodate their needs.

"They were essentially trying to wait it out and get themselves better," Godbold said.

In ongoing legal action against the prison system, Godbold's firm claims Donovan guards have physically abused disabled inmates and then denied them medical care, leaving some too scared to seek help when they need it. About a quarter of people incarcerated at Donovan are disabled.

Godbold said her firm's reports show about half of the 219 state prisoners who have died from COVID-19 had disabilities.

"These are serious red flags," she said.

Kenneth Sandlin, a Donovan prisoner found dead in his cell, tested negative for the virus almost three weeks before his death, medical examiner records show. He refused to be tested again even after developing a persistent cough.

On December 27, Sandlin told his cellmate he wasn't feeling well and went to sleep on the top bunk. That afternoon, staff found the 65-year-old unresponsive and attempted CPR. They took him to the triage department, where he was pronounced dead.

The Medical Examiner's Office tested Sandlin's body and found he was positive for the virus.

Sandlin, who was serving a 25-year sentence for voluntary manslaughter, had cirrhosis, according to medical examiner records. That put him at an increased risk of complications from the coronavirus.

Incarcerated people have higher rates of many medical conditions, making them more susceptible to developing serious symptoms and dying from COVID-19. Prisons are also hotbeds for outbreaks because confined quarters and low airflow enable the virus to spread quickly.

The state corrections system began vaccinating inmates in December, but vaccines weren't introduced at Donovan until after the worst of its outbreak had passed and inmates were already dead. As of this week, 73% of incarcerated people and 44% of staff are fully vaccinated. There is one active COVID-19 case.

Advocates say vaccinations in prisons are also essential to fighting the virus in the community. Research has linked high COVID-19 infection levels inside prisons to increased cases in neighboring areas.

Aviram, the UC Hastings law professor, said even though people imagine prisons as walled-off facilities, they operate more like membranes, with staff, volunteers and inmates leaving and entering each day. The activity puts the surrounding neighborhoods at risk.

"All of this enormous effort that everybody's been putting forth in the last year, social distancing and masking and doing without and sacrificing," she said, "all of this stuff is going to be worthless if we continue to incubate this disease in a place where hundreds of people go in and out on a regular basis."

Inewsource intern Kate Sequeira contributed to this story

Jill Castellano and Mary Plummer
Donovan Deaths: Families Kept in Dark While Inmates Die of COVID-19

This story was originally produced and published by inewsource, a nonprofit, nonpartisan newsroom in San Diego committed to exposing wrongdoing and holding powerful people and institutions accountable. As part of their commitment to keeping the San Diego community informed, inewsource has allowed this story to be reprinted and shared here with you. To learn more about their work and how you can support their journalism, visit inewsource.org.

April 9, 2021

He died on Christmas Day, four months shy of his first parole hearing after more than 20 years in prison.

Earlie Paton was incarcerated at Richard J. Donovan Correctional Facility in Otay Mesa when he tested positive for COVID-19 in December. His breathing grew shallow, so the prison sent him to a nearby hospital.

The 67-year-old's condition only got worse over four days at UC San Diego Medical Center. He chose to withdraw from treatment and died the next day.

Paton's family says they weren't told about his death for about a month.

Two of his siblings, Byron Porter and Candice Fleming, said they were shocked to learn the news. Their brother was scheduled for a parole hearing in April. They were looking forward to his possible release.

"They didn't tell us he was sick. They didn't tell us nothing," Porter said, calling the death an "injustice."

The state corrections department said it notified Paton's registered next of kin within 72 hours of his death, and those not on the list wouldn't be told right away.

Porter maintains that did not happen, and his siblings should have been contacted while their brother was alive, so they could have said goodbye.

Paton was one of 18 people incarcerated at Donovan to die from COVID-19 during a winter outbreak. The prison is among the most deadly in the state: It is tied for the third highest death count from the virus. Roughly 30% of people serving sentences there have contracted COVID-19 during the pandemic.

The deceased were as young as 48 and as old as 83. More than half were Black, Hispanic, or Native American. At least 14 had underlying medical conditions. Three were found unresponsive in their cells, while others were taken to hospitals before their deaths.

Inewsource interviewed the families of five inmates who died. Their stories had one thing in common: No prison officials alerted them their loved ones were seriously ill until after their deaths.

California Department of Corrections and Rehabilitation spokespeople have refused to provide reporters with any specifics about the inmates' illnesses or deaths, citing health privacy laws like HIPAA. The details included in this story were gathered from an extensive review of San Diego County medical examiner reports, legal proceedings, death certificates and interviews with the people close to those who died.

Together, they reveal a disturbing picture of a prison system that prioritizes privacy over transparency in life and death.

A third of the prisoners who died weren't diagnosed with COVID-19 until they were taken to a hospital, despite federal guidance around frequent virus testing. Six withdrew from treatment while hospitalized, yet some of their families say they still weren't told their loved ones were near death. And the relatives of four incarcerated men said once they were notified of the deaths, the prison refused to answer many questions about medical care or conditions inside the facility.

"It's a dereliction of duty," said Sharon Dolovich, a UCLA law professor and director of a national project that tracks COVID-19 in jails and prisons, when learning of inewsource's findings. "It's gross inhumanity. And it just reflects the system that does not see the people in its custody as human beings who have family members and loved ones."

The corrections department is supposed to inform emergency contacts when an inmate becomes seriously ill. But because of safety and security concerns, a spokesperson said, it doesn't always follow that policy when someone is transported to a hospital.

Marcus Pollard, the warden at Donovan prison, declined multiple interview requests through a spokesperson.

"This American obsession with medical privacy and with HIPAA becomes this blanket that hides all matters of atrocities that are happening under the guise that you're protecting the privacy of the patients," said Hadar Aviram, a criminologist and professor at the UC Hastings College of Law in San Francisco.

"The inhumanity is shocking," she added.

Life-Saving Measures

Donovan inmate Elmer Lee, an Army veteran who served in Vietnam, was hospitalized twice in the month before his death. The prison didn't tell his son until after Lee opted to withdraw from treatment and died.

Robert Lee spoke with his father about a week before his death. He said the 74-year-old was in great spirits, despite his leukemia and other ongoing health conditions. When he got a call from the prison with the news, he said he was "dumbfounded."

He thinks his father would have wanted to speak with him before transitioning to do-not-resuscitate status.

"I knew he was having the medical issues, but it was like running into a wall in a dark room," Lee said.

Elmer Lee died of cardiovascular disease, with COVID-19 as a contributing factor.

"To find out he passed away, it just floored me," his son said.

Lee was serving a life sentence with the possibility of parole for sexual abuse of a child under 14 and other related offenses.

The prison system's process for notifying the family of inmates when they become gravely ill or die can be convoluted and bureaucratic.

Inmates are asked to update a form annually with emergency contacts who are supposed to be notified of any serious illnesses and injuries, as well as after death. But a state prison spokesperson said families aren't told when their loved ones are taken to a hospital, though exceptions are made if a medical surrogate is needed.

After learning of his father's death, Robert Lee faced months of confusing phone calls to try to collect any remaining personal items, which he still hasn't received. He also wasn't prepared to pay the almost $1,000 in cremation costs for his father's remains—something advocates argue the prison system should pay for—and had to set up a monthly payment plan with the funeral home.

The one thing Lee wishes the prison system had done differently was given him a chance to say goodbye to his father.

"What would have been nice is being able to talk to him while he was in the hospital," his son said.

Staff at each of California's 35 adult prisons are tasked with notifying next of kin within 72 hours of an inmate's death, according to the department's 840-page operations manual. A spokesperson said that protocol was followed for all those at Donovan who died from the coronavirus.

Lee was told about his father's death the same day it happened. In cases where family members aren't registered as emergency contacts, it can take much longer.

The prison system says it uses all resources possible to track down a contact when none is listed. If it can't find one, the Medical Examiner's Office takes over and conducts a search for any possible relatives to give them the chance to collect the remains.

In the case of Earlie Paton, the corrections department didn't have next-of-kin information when it notified the medical examiner of his death on Christmas. The office's investigators began a search for his relatives the next day.

It took two weeks for the office to learn the prison had found Paton's family, and then another 10 days before learning all of his nine living siblings had been reached.

The state corrections department said the person listed as next of kin in Paton's records was contacted within 72 hours of his death, but it wouldn't say who that was. Porter, his brother, believes he was listed as the contact but didn't find out about Paton's death for weeks.

When he finally received the call from a corrections staffer about his brother's death, the news was more confusing than anything. He thought Paton was hundreds of miles away at another institution. Nobody had told him his brother had been transferred from Corcoran state prison in Central California to Donovan in October, two months before he died.

The corrections department wouldn't explain why Paton was transferred in the middle of the pandemic, despite federal guidelines discouraging the movement of prisoners between facilities to curb the spread of COVID-19.

"He has a son, a family that cared about him, a family that loved him," said Fleming, Paton's sister. "We just want to know what happened to our brother."

Paton was sentenced to life in prison in 1998 for two counts of indecent exposure with prior felony convictions. His family felt the prison system punished him for his mental illness, called exhibitionism, which involves showing one's genitals to nonconsenting people.

Prison officials had disciplined Paton 10 times for indecent exposure since 2016. In September, the state extended his sentence by eight months because of the offenses. Paton also had a previous conviction for indecent exposure in Los Angeles County, which resulted in a two-year prison term.

"They're doing those prisoners so terrible," Fleming said. "It needs to be totally reformed."

A Death Sentence

Federal guidelines encourage prisons to perform widespread testing during COVID-19 outbreaks so they can isolate those who are sick, prevent future infections, and ensure the ill get the care they need.

At the height of Donovan's winter outbreak, more than 700 incarcerated people contracted the virus, one of the highest infection rates across the state at the time.

Corrections officials maintain that inmates were tested at the prison weekly in December and January. But six Donovan prisoners who died during the outbreak weren't diagnosed with COVID-19 until they were transported to the hospital, according to medical examiner reports.

No available records suggest any of them were tested before being hospitalized.

One of them, 56-year-old Paul Martinez, was sick for six days at Donovan with some of the most common COVID-19 symptoms—shortness of breath, fever, and coughing. Records show the diagnosis came at the hospital, when he arrived with shallow breathing.

Another, Duane Everly, was diagnosed with COVID-19 at Alvarado hospital in early January, where he was sent for care because he was short of breath. Doctors provided the 51-year-old with oxygen and medication, but it didn't work. Everly died on January 7.

His uncle, Darnell Everly, said the prison told him his nephew started complaining about COVID-19 symptoms in the few days before he died.

"That's what got me curious," he said, explaining he thought the symptoms took longer than that to manifest. But the Donovan employee he spoke with would tell him little about his nephew's medical condition and would not say how many others at the facility were infected.

Lawyers at the Prison Law Office, which represents inmates at California correctional facilities, were able to access Everly's medical records. In a court filing, they say prison doctors ordered COVID-19 tests for Everly three times in December, but none were performed.

The law office reviewed medical records for more than 20 Donovan inmates and concluded "the prison had many, perhaps hundreds of orders for COVID-19 testing in December that had apparently not been done, timely or otherwise."

The corrections department has denied in court filings issues with access to coronavirus tests.

Everly was one of at least seven Donovan inmates to die from COVID-19 who had had their prison terms lengthened under California's three-strikes law, which mandates long sentences for those with previous violent or serious felony convictions.

The Arizona native lived in group homes throughout his childhood. He was medicated for auditory hallucinations by the time he was 10. By 18, he was bouncing between the streets and staying with his grandmother in Pomona.

That's when he committed his first-strike offense, in 1987, when he stole a woman's purse. He was convicted of second-degree robbery. Everly didn't face another serious conviction until 2019, when he faced two counts of assault with intent to commit a sex offense.

His defense attorneys said he was offered an eight-year deal but maintained his innocence and wanted to go to trial.

When he was convicted, they argued that because more than 30 years had passed since his first strike, he should receive a lighter prison term. They were stunned when the judge sentenced him to 29 years—far longer than they had seen other clients receive in more serious cases.

"He needed help, not to be put in prison where he was ultimately given a de facto death sentence," said Dan Kapelovitz, a Los Angeles criminal defense attorney who represented Everly in the trial.

Everly's family is holding a service for him Friday in Phoenix. His father's grave will be opened so that his ashes can be spread on top.

Kapelovitz kept in touch with Everly as he continued to appeal his sentence. He and his co-counsel, Ted Batsakis, still remember Everly's kindness and sense of humor. They said he never showed any signs of a violent temperament.

"The man was willing to do his time," Batsakis said. "And God willing, he would have done his time and gotten out, maybe had a few years left to live a good life as best as he could. That's the sad part here."

Among the Dead

The Donovan inmates who died from COVID-19 were incarcerated on a range of charges. Some were serving time for high-profile cases that spawned documentaries or books.

After a heated trial, Robert Peernock, an 83-year-old from Los Angeles, was imprisoned for the murder of his estranged wife and attempted murder of his daughter in 1987. Leon Martinez, 48, was convicted in a cold case murder solved in 2006 with the help of new DNA technology.

Samuel Baca Duran was sentenced to life without the possibility of parole for murdering his ex-wife in 2001. He died in Alvarado hospital's intensive care unit on December 27.

Donna Duran, the couple's daughter, said it took time for her to process her father's death. She hadn't seen or spoken to him since his sentencing but agreed to collect his remains and have him cremated.

"It's complete closure," she said.

Regardless of their crimes, advocates and public health experts contend prisoners did not have to die from COVID-19.

Dolovich and her team at UCLA have spent the pandemic tracking down data on COVID-19's impact in detention centers, hoping to help prevent similar outbreaks in the future. They publish a scorecard rating the transparency of correctional facilities across the U.S. and the ease of access to COVID-19 data. California's prison system scored a C.

"What's come out during the pandemic is the way in which corrections officials are somehow confused and think that the information about what happens in the prison is proprietary to them," Dolovich said.

"Prison officials are not sovereign," she added. "They are public servants."

Jill Castellano and Mary Plummer
First COVID-19 Wrongful Death Claim Filed by Family of Donovan Inmate

> *This story was originally produced and published by inewsource, a nonprofit, nonpartisan newsroom in San Diego committed to exposing wrongdoing and holding powerful people and institutions accountable. As part of their commitment to keeping the San Diego community informed, inewsource has allowed this story to be reprinted and shared here with you. To learn more about their work and how you can support their journalism, visit inewsource.org.*

May 25, 2021

The family of a man incarcerated in San Diego who died from COVID-19 has filed a wrongful death claim against the California corrections department.

The claim, submitted to the Office of Insurance and Risk Management on May 9, is a precursor to filing a lawsuit against the state for its role in Leon Martinez's death.

It is the only known claim that has been filed against the San Diego prison for a COVID-19 death, the risk management office said, and one of seven that has been filed across the state prison system.

Martinez was serving a sentence of 28 years to life in prison at the Richard J. Donovan Correctional Facility in Otay Mesa for his role in a high-profile cold case murder. At 48, he was the youngest of 18 Donovan inmates to die from the virus.

Martinez's wife and three children allege staff refused to wear masks or engage in social distancing, leading him to contract COVID-19. Once he was sick, the claim says, he was not given the medical care he needed.

The filing also describes that Donovan inmates with COVID-19 were kept in close quarters with those who were not infected, which prison officials have acknowledged took place during a winter outbreak.

Hospital records show Martinez had a myriad of underlying medical conditions—including asthma, uncontrolled diabetes, hepatitis C, anemia, and seizure disorder—that can increase the chances of COVID-19 complications.

Evangelina Garcia, Martinez's wife, said the prison should have identified him as high-risk when the pandemic began and moved him to a clean and secure housing area where he would not have contracted the virus.

"They're accountable for what happened to him," said Garcia, who lives in Yucaipa in San Bernardino County. "I feel they let us down. I feel they gave him a life sentence he was not supposed to have."

By coincidence, Garcia had COVID-19 in December, at the same time as her husband, but she quickly recovered from her fever and chills. Martinez never did.

"This isn't the way it was supposed to end," Garcia said.

A spokesperson for the corrections department would not answer questions about Martinez's death or his family's claim, citing health privacy laws and a policy to not comment on pending litigation. The department has previously defended its response to the pandemic, pointing to vastly reduced infection rates in state prisons, and said it takes the health and safety of its residents seriously.

The prison system has said medical staff regularly monitor COVID-positive inmates and transfer them to hospitals if they need a higher level of care.

Martinez died in the wake of a massive winter outbreak at Donovan prison that resulted in 700 infections, 18 inmate deaths and one staff death. Statewide, nearly 50,000 California prisoners have contracted the virus and more than 200 have died.

Martinez was convicted of killing 17-year-old Victoria Ghonim, a crime that occurred in 1992 while her infant son was in the car. The case went unsolved for more than a decade, but when investigators tested DNA from the scene in 2006, they matched it to Martinez and his roommate. Martinez later testified that the victim's husband offered to pay him $20,000 to commit the murder, though the dollar figure has been disputed in court. He was convicted in 2015.

Garcia was also sentenced in the case. She served three months in jail for attempting to discourage Martinez's ex-girlfriend from testifying against him.

Martinez's family said his crime and conviction didn't change the way they viewed him or how much they loved him. His children were looking forward to his possible release from prison in 2029.

"He was my best friend. He was my everything," his son Andrew Martinez said.

Since his mother was diagnosed with colon cancer in 2016, Andrew and his father have spoken on the phone almost every day.

The 19-year-old said the claim will help the family hold the prison accountable for his father's death.

"We all would've felt bad if we just let it happen," he said.

Calling for Answers

Garcia knew something was wrong when Leon Martinez didn't call on their daughter's birthday like he did every year. The next day, on his own birthday—New Year's Eve of 2020—the phone still didn't ring.

As the days passed, the family grew more concerned. Martinez had rarely been out of touch for that long in his 12 years behind bars. On

January 8, Garcia tried calling at least eight phone numbers for Donovan with no success. A prison counselor finally told her Martinez had been transferred to a hospital, but he wouldn't say which hospital or why.

Medical records show Martinez tested positive for COVID-19 at Donovan on January 5. The prison called 911 two days later because he had trouble breathing.

When he arrived at Alvarado Hospital Medical Center in eastern San Diego, Martinez had a dangerously low blood oxygen level of 77% and was treated for respiratory failure. He was transferred to the intensive care unit that day and diagnosed with pneumonia.

Meanwhile, Garcia was calling hospitals throughout San Diego County searching for her husband. When she finally learned he was at Alvarado, she said she left her phone number with hospital staff, but nobody would tell her about Martinez's condition.

On January 11, his fever rose to 103 degrees, and he was placed on a ventilator. That's when a doctor at Donovan called Garcia to explain her husband had COVID-19 and it was serious. The staff member wouldn't answer many of her questions, Garcia said.

Without permission from the hospital or prison, Garcia immediately drove to Alvarado. Healthcare staff wouldn't allow her in Martinez's room, but they did let her see him on a video call.

Alvarado hospital did not answer questions about Martinez's illness and death or its protocols for treating incarcerated patients.

For the following two weeks, the family was left to wait.

"It was just torture for us," Garcia said.

After days of incessant calling, a Donovan doctor told Garcia her husband's condition had not changed—he remained on a ventilator with COVID-19—and said the prison would only call back if Martinez died.

On January 23, Garcia received a call from the prison saying her husband was in critical condition and that she could visit him in the hospital. When she arrived with Martinez's three children, the family was not allowed to speak to him and could only peer at his medical bed across the room through a glass window. They could barely see his face.

Leon Martinez Jr., 22, said it was the first time he had seen his father since his conviction seven years earlier. The trauma of visiting his father in county jail before being transferred to prison—shackled and prevented from hugging—kept him away from the correctional facility. This time, his father was unconscious and hooked up to a ventilator.

"I just felt like, I don't know. It felt unreal," he said.

A day after the visit, Martinez crashed. Medics performed CPR but couldn't revive him. He died on January 25.

"It breaks my heart because he was robbed of being there for his kids," said Martinez's first wife, Sunshine Martinez.

"He has a lot of people that really love him and will always love him," she added.

Born in Los Angeles County, Martinez had his first son, Leon Jr., with Sunshine Martinez in 1998. The couple divorced and Martinez moved to Yucaipa, where he met and married Garcia. They had a son and daughter together, and when they could get away from work, they would take the children camping, riding ATVs, and exploring the wilderness.

Martinez's family described him as an outgoing man and supportive father. He was never able to meet his 4-year-old grandson, Leon Martinez III.

Martinez Jr. said his father turned him into a fly fisher and outdoorsman who is almost always by the river or in the mountains.

"When I'm out there, I feel so good, like I'm with my dad," he said.

In those moments, he said, the grief of his father's unexpected death fades away.

"I Still Need Answers"

An inewsource investigation in April found at least five people incarcerated at Donovan died from COVID-19 before their families knew they were sick.

The corrections department requires inmates to have multiple forms on file if their relatives want updates on their medical conditions. Even with the paperwork complete, the prison system has said it usually doesn't tell families about inmate hospitalizations for security reasons.

Garcia said her husband had filled out the necessary forms, and she should have received clearer communication about his illness. She said Martinez was strongly opposed to being ventilated, but she was not given a chance to relay that to his doctors or help guide his medical care.

A corrections department spokesperson did not respond to questions about what happened in the weeks before Martinez died.

A case summary written by an Alvarado hospital doctor on January 25 says Martinez was "ripping his lines and broke a high flow oxygen machine" before he was placed on a ventilator. Later that day, when doctors inserted a catheter into his neck, medical notes described it as an emergency procedure and that there was "no family available" to consent.

Donovan has released little information about the incarcerated people and staff member who died from COVID-19. Garcia said nobody has told her how Martinez contracted the virus or what medical care he received before he was taken to the hospital.

"I still need answers and accountability," Garcia said.

Almost two months after Martinez died, Garcia and her son Andrew drove almost two hours to Donovan to pick up Martinez's belongings. The boxes were lighter than they expected, and when they opened one up, they couldn't believe it. The prison had given them a different inmate's property, Garcia said.

They drove back to the prison and were able to get the correct items. The relatives of three other Donovan inmates who died from COVID-19 told inewsource they are still waiting to receive their loved ones' belongings more than four months after their deaths.

"We felt very disrespected," Garcia said. "That was the last thing they could have made right. They had their chance to make that right for us."

A corrections department spokesperson said Donovan prison is reviewing its property handling process as a result of the mix-up with Martinez's belongings.

Donovan's Track Record

Legal filings and administrative reports show Donovan has among the worst track records of California's 35 adult prisons for its handling of the pandemic. In an ongoing class action case, the prison acknowledged housing COVID-positive inmates with people who didn't have the virus because employees were overwhelmed by the winter outbreak.

The state's prison oversight office found Donovan issued its staff with the most written citations of any prison for refusing to wear masks or practice social distancing in December—around the time when Martinez and hundreds of others contracted the virus.

A new report the oversight office released on May 19 found the corrections department has done a poor job controlling problem prison staff around the state. It paid out more than $1 million in salaries and benefits to employees in the past two years while moving slowly on their discipline cases.

"I don't think Mr. Martinez's case is an isolated case whatsoever," said civil rights attorney Salomon Zavala, who filed the family's claim.

He called the prison's treatment of Martinez and other Donovan inmates "a deliberate indifference of the life of these individuals that were incarcerated."

Zavala said attorneys are often reluctant to take on complex wrongful death lawsuits on behalf of prisoners—the payouts can be low and take years to manifest—but he chose to work on Martinez's case after hearing the family's story.

"This case reeks of the lack of humanity," Zavala said.

Few COVID-19 wrongful death cases have been brought so far against the California corrections department. The family of San Quentin inmate Daniel Ruiz sued the prison system in federal court in March, alleging a botched transfer of inmates from another state prison led to widespread infections and Ruiz's death.

Of the seven known COVID-19 wrongful death claims against the state prison system, the Martinez family's claim is the only one still under review—five others were rejected by the risk management office, and one was incomplete.

Bringing a lawsuit against the California government is a multi-year process that has grown longer during the pandemic. Because of the state's COVID-19 executive order, the period to file a wrongful death claim has been extended to one year, and the office has about six months to review it.

If the Martinez family's claim is rejected, they can sue. The lawsuit could take five or more years to be resolved because of a growing backlog of court cases.

Garcia said she hopes her actions will help other families affected by COVID-19 deaths at Donovan who may not know how to file a claim or advocate for change in the prison system.

"Every inmate there either has a mother, a father, a son, a daughter, a wife praying for them out here," she said. "And we're doing the time with them."

covid-19 hotels

Cody Dulaney
San Diego County Won't Provide 24/7 Medical Services at COVID-19 Hotels, Despite SDSU Advice

> *This story was originally produced and published by inewsource, a nonprofit, nonpartisan newsroom in San Diego committed to exposing wrongdoing and holding powerful people and institutions accountable. As part of their commitment to keeping the San Diego community informed, inewsource has allowed this story to be reprinted and shared here with you. To learn more about their work and how you can support their journalism, visit inewsource.org.*

October 1, 2021

San Diego County officials insist they've already fixed most of the problems outlined in a scathing independent review of the county's COVID hotel sheltering program.

And despite recommendations from San Diego State University, officials said they will not provide around-the-clock nurses, mental health services, or over-the-counter medications for people isolating in the hotels.

County staff told the Board of Supervisors that those changes are not necessary "based on the current hotel population, and the infrequent requests for services," according to a seven-page memo dated September 29. Staff will move to implement those changes if needed, the memo said.

The hotel program, established in March 2020, was the first of its kind in an attempt to prevent the spread of COVID-19. It was intended to provide temporary housing for those who needed somewhere to isolate after coming in contact with the virus—many of whom are homeless and might be struggling with mental illness or substance-use disorders—and has now served more than 12,000 people. But it has been plagued with problems from the beginning.

The memo, obtained by inewsource Thursday, is in response to a commissioned SDSU evaluation that confirmed inewsource reporting over the past year and a half about neglect and mismanagement in the troubled hotel program.

Released August 3, the evaluation commended county staff for successfully preventing the spread. But it also said the county's contractor, Equus Workforce Solutions, is unqualified to run the program and employs poorly trained staff, who forced residents to suffer through long delays for much-needed medication and who allowed gaps in services that may have led to overdoses and suicide.

The memo is the county's first indication of what officials are doing to improve the hotel program, but it only addresses the first of SDSU's nine recommendations—the one that suggests 14 changes to improve the program right away.

The need for on-site nurses, behavioral health specialists, and access to over-the-counter medicine 24 hours a day was at the top of SDSU's list of suggested changes. But since SDSU's evaluation, officials have said the program had to pivot from assisting mainly homeless people with COVID-19 to asylum seekers released by Customs and Border Protection, meaning this new population has different needs.

According to the memo, county officials said they have already addressed nine of those suggested changes and implemented quality assurance measures. That includes ensuring medications are delivered in a reasonable amount of time, offering unlimited snacks and water, assigning one case manager to coordinate services for each guest, and providing clean bedding, towels, and toilet paper in a timely manner.

Officials have also taken steps to fix two other problems: Improve the food selection and delivery, and ensure staff follows a script for intake calls, wellness checks, or other screening services.

But they rejected three other recommendations. In addition to 24/7 medical services, officials also declined to limit deliveries and search people's belongings, unless there's a safety issue. That recommendation stemmed from rampant drug use that has occurred in the hotels.

This plan of action comes one week after a county spokesperson described an expanding program and an elevated need for services to justify an $83 million payment increase for Equus in the middle of the evaluation. Staff wanted to ensure funding is available as quickly as possible in case of a pending surge in cases, a spokesperson said. All told, the county is on track to spend $140.6 million, with Equus providing invoices for services provided.

The County Board of Supervisors ordered the evaluation in early March, after an inewsource investigation exposed severe gaps in services and a suicide in a hotel room that wasn't discovered for five days. Officials agreed to pay SDSU $140,000 for the evaluation but have refused to answer specific questions about the findings.

Inewsource has attempted to interview every county board member since release of the report, but none have been willing to discuss it in an interview.

In a statement released Friday, Board Chairman Nathan Fletcher said county officials and contract employees have had to respond quickly to an unprecedented pandemic. They continue to take action when unpredictable situations arise and make improvements as needed.

"My request for the independent evaluation of services at the isolation hotel was an acknowledgment that improvements to the services were necessary," Fletcher said. "Fortunately, our county team and contractors did not wait for the final report to begin making some of the improvements."

Hundreds of people will continue relying on services at these hotels until the county's contract with Equus expires at the end of the year. As of now, there are no plans to discuss the report or the future of the program at a public meeting.

Healthcare and Wrap-Around Services

At the COVID-19 hotels, access to nurses, mental health specialists, and medication is only available from 7 a.m. to 11:30 p.m., even though hotel guests are under a public health order to stay in their rooms while many suffer through COVID-19 symptoms.

But the county contends that the program is only supposed to provide a place to isolate and does not need "hospital-level care." That underscores one of SDSU's findings—a disagreement among county officials about the type of program that is needed. Some said the goal was simply to isolate people and prevent community spread. But others recognized that these hotels would become a shelter serving primarily vulnerable people with complex needs.

SDSU seems to agree that additional help is necessary, as four of the nine recommendations listed in the report deal with case management and medical or behavioral health services. The report goes on to say that all similar programs in the future should focus on medical and behavioral health services.

But "the most significant complaint" dealt with long delays for over-the-counter medications, SDSU's report said.

"In several instances, the guest was ill with COVID-19, exhibiting symptoms such as fever, aches, chills, diarrhea, headaches, and vomiting, but experienced long delays in receiving medications."

One guest told SDSU researchers, "I had diarrhea and was vomiting, but I had to wait for medication. If I asked for it in the middle of the night, I would not get it until the next morning."

Even on day shifts, SDSU said, several guests were forced to wait hours for medications.

Despite that, county officials don't feel it's necessary at this time to provide access to medication 24-hours a day. Medications are typically delivered within 30 minutes of request, the memo said, and officials will implement a quality assurance process to adhere to that timeline. But if the need arises, staff will find a contractor to make it work.

Until then, a spokesperson said the county has established a process to ensure people are provided doses to cover them through overnight shifts.

Mental health services were also identified as a weakness in SDSU's report. The county has a contract with Telecare Corp. worth $13 million to provide that support, but a county staff member said, "Telecare is behavioral health lite. It is not for acute care. It can't be used for crisis stabilization."

Equus employees told SDSU they had only received on-the-job training, and never received formal training on behavioral health, trauma-informed care, or de-escalation techniques. According to county staff, that has since changed. Equus now requires those trainings, as well as cultural diversity and conflict resolution. Officials did not say when that change was made.

Case managers are responsible for connecting people with the services they need, whether it's housing, financial assistance, substance abuse, or mental health, and SDSU found some of that work was happening. The majority of people experiencing homelessness before entering the program returned to another shelter setting, while 22 people moved into permanent supportive housing, which was considered "an impressive accomplishment," the report said.

But no single person is assigned to a guest to oversee all aspects of their care. Instead, the services are provided piecemeal, and responsibilities are divided among multiple staff members.

"These gaps in care coordination may have led to both overdoses and suicide," one county staff member said.

This has been addressed, too, according to the memo. Each guest is assigned to a social support counselor to coordinate services, but officials haven't said whether each guest will have one person coordinating all aspects of care or when that change was made.

Hygiene and Food Quality

Most of the guests who responded to a survey had positive comments about the program, but some described uncomfortable and harrowing experiences during SDSU interviews.

"Employees treat us like animals, without any compassion," a pregnant woman with two kids wrote in a complaint after leaving the program, according to the report.

"I don't want any family to go through what I went through. It's all inhumane," she added.

Several guests said they needed clean sheets and towels but were told they were not available, or they would have to be placed on a waiting list, the SDSU report said.

"I cried myself to sleep because of being very sick and worried I would die," one person told SDSU. "I could not get new bedding or towels—they said they couldn't do it—not even drop me off some. I had been sweating in them for days. I had to dry the towels on the AC unit. When I asked for towels, they told me that this was not like regular hotel service."

Others complained about not having any toilet paper, with one guest saying they had to get into the shower to clean up each time they used the toilet.

But now, county staff said all rooms are cleaned and restocked with bedding and towels prior to check-in, and that guests may use the room phone to request more. On average, items are provided within 30 minutes, and officials will rely on guest satisfaction surveys to quickly address any areas that need improvement. Officials have not said when those changes were implemented.

A spokesperson said providing these necessities has always been a priority, and while SDSU identified instances when this goal was not met, "the suggestion that it was a universal experience is not accurate."

Guests also complained about being refused snacks and water, despite the county's contention that an unlimited supply has always been available upon request. But now, a quality assurance guest satisfaction survey will be used to gauge whether this is happening, according to the county's memo.

Food quality was a big issue for hotel guests. Many complained they were hungry and portion sizes were too small. Some told SDSU they went hungry because they were repeatedly given meals they were allergic to or couldn't eat, and they were told their needs couldn't be met.

To fix that, county officials said Equus is "actively pursuing options to provide additional choices for meals," and even started a pilot program last month to provide two additional dinner options. The county will rely on surveys to address any issues in the future, the memo said.

County officials plan to use SDSU's report "as a valuable tool for identifying areas of continued refinement" for this program, as well as all similar programs in the future.

A spokesperson said the other eight recommendations listed in SDSU's report—one of which includes evaluating the other Equus-run hotels for medically-compromised people who have nowhere to isolate—will be considered in the future.

Jill Castellano contributed to this report

Cody Dulaney and Jill Castellano

Problems Plague COVID-19 Hotel After County Pays Company Millions to Run It

This story was originally produced and published by inewsource, a nonprofit, nonpartisan newsroom in San Diego committed to exposing wrongdoing and holding powerful people and institutions accountable. As part of their commitment to keeping the San Diego community informed, inewsource has allowed this story to be reprinted and shared here with you. To learn more about their work and how you can support their journalism, visit inewsource.org.

February 22, 2021

Two months after inewsource reported a spike in police calls, a lapse in mental healthcare, and a suicide death at a COVID-19 isolation hotel, San Diego County shifted the operation of its sheltering program to a staffing agency for $30 million.

But problems at the Crowne Plaza hotel in Mission Valley appear to be no better today.

Hotel guests and employees told inewsource the program is mismanaged, staff aren't properly trained, and security guards harass those who are under a public health order to isolate. It's all causing some to leave the hotel before they're supposed to.

Records show the high volume of police calls to the Crowne Plaza has also continued, as have reports of suicide threats and overdoses.

"They're shooting from the hip," said Turquoise Teagle, a site coordinator at the hotel who works for the county's contractor, Equus Workforce Solutions.

"I think the county should come in, revamp the program, and get Equus out of there, honestly."

Teagle, 35, said she was placed on paid administrative leave after repeatedly complaining to her supervisors about the poor care at the hotel. Among the problems she said she's reported:

- Guests don't receive their medication on time, and children have gone days without appropriate food.
- Employees aren't told how and when to coordinate with Telecare Corp., which the county pays to provide mental and behavioral health services.
- Staff aren't prepared to work with most of those who are isolating—people who are homeless and might be struggling with mental illness or substance-use disorders.

Another employee described similar conditions but fears being fired so inewsource agreed not to name them.

Neither Equus employee inewsource interviewed said they had seen county officials visit the hotel. County officials get their information from daily video meetings, where an Equus supervisor reads updates to faces on a computer screen.

A former Crowne Plaza guest, William Morris, who stayed there in November with his wife after she tested positive for COVID-19, said a dispute about his service dog escalated to a security guard attempting to hit him with a chair.

"I wouldn't put my worst enemy in a place like that," Morris said, adding that security was his biggest issue. "They don't have empathy for people, compassion for people, and they're a bunch of animals running wild."

When the pandemic began last March, the county took over the Crowne Plaza and other hotels to temporarily house people who needed somewhere to stay. The goal was twofold: To isolate people who test positive or come in contact with the virus, and to protect people who are at risk for developing severe illness.

The county has refused to identify all the facilities in use, citing privacy concerns for the people in isolation, but said about 950 rooms have been secured.

County spokesperson Michael Workman said in emails to inewsource that officials are in daily communication with contractors, conduct site visits at least once a month, and are notified of any serious incidents. He added that Equus has received "several positive comments from guests at Crowne Plaza" in satisfaction surveys.

As for the frequent police presence at the hotel, Workman said on-site security is supposed to "monitor any situations which may require law enforcement involvement."

"Some of the individuals we have provided isolation for also have a high degree of behavioral health needs," he said. "In addition, the impact of isolation and the challenges with addressing the pandemic often contribute to an increase in behavioral health symptoms."

Despite that, Teagle said Equus never provided any mental health training, and she had no idea what to expect when she started her job.

"I feel like speaking out on it will just bring more attention to it, and maybe the county will be a little bit more hands-on with everything that's going on," Teagle said.

"How Do You Not Realize That?"

Early in the pandemic, county staff operating the Crowne Plaza became overwhelmed.

An employee overseeing operations sent an email March 26 to colleagues saying she was "pushing and begging and pleading for additional staff" to help with the workload, "and to provide adequate support to the folks in the hotels."

Within a week, county officials changed an existing $13 million contract it had with Telecare, which had been providing mental health services to San Diegans in the legal system, to also help people in isolation.

But it didn't make a difference for 28-year-old Jose Angel Gomez-Camacho. He died by suicide at the Crowne Plaza three weeks later.

Gomez-Camacho was living on the streets, diagnosed with schizophrenia, and addicted to crystal meth when county officials placed him at the hotel, according to his brother, Jorge Gomez.

Gomez, 31, said he and his younger brother, Jose, grew up poor in San Diego County. They had a rough childhood, he said, and they followed different paths.

"My brother took more of a liking to the streets. I tried to live my life as best as I could," Gomez said.

His brother struggled with addiction for years, and family members think that's what led to his mental illness. The last time family saw him was on his birthday in early April. He tested positive for the virus soon after and was sent to the Crowne Plaza.

County employees are supposed to check on each guest once a day. But after Jose tested negative for the virus, "it was presumed he left the hotel," county medical examiner records show.

Five days passed before hotel staff found him on April 23.

"How do you not realize that there's somebody dead in your hotel? How do you not realize that?" Gomez said.

He believes San Diego County should bear some responsibility for what happened to his brother.

If he had been given the care he needed, Gomez said, "we wouldn't be having this conversation right now."

Workman, the county spokesperson, said he could not comment on the specifics of the case because of privacy concerns but explained "there was an incident where a guest was able to gain reentry to a room after check-out." Staff didn't know the guest was there because they thought the room was empty, he said.

The medical examiner's records on Jose's death weren't public while the county investigated what happened, but they were recently released to inewsource. The county would not answer questions about its investigation.

"It wasn't easy for me to process this," Gomez said. "There's times where I blame myself, and I have to stop doing it because it's getting nowhere."

A $30 Million Contract

Two months after Jose's death, San Diego County asked Equus to run its COVID-19 sheltering program. Officials realized the staffing agency can "perform the services more economically and efficiently than the county," according to the contract signed on July 1.

Equus is responsible for providing guests with three meals a day, laundry services, on-site security, and medications, relying on several subcontractors to get the job done. Equus employees also arrange transportation to and from the hotel, screen people to assess their needs for healthcare and government benefits, and work on discharge plans, either into permanent housing or another shelter.

The county paid Equus $10.2 million in 2020. If services are needed through the end of this year, it will cost an additional $20 million.

While Equus oversees the daily operations, Telecare is still responsible for providing mental and behavioral health services at the county-run hotels. Since August, Telecare has received more than $350,000 for its work at the hotels through funding the county received under the federal CARES Act.

Public records show Telecare has a history of not fulfilling its duties. In the past six years, the company had to issue corrective action plans for at least four contracts it held in California.

That includes an incident in 2015, in which Telecare decided not to bill Los Angeles County for $153,000 in services it was supposed to have provided. The company said "leadership vacancies" had caused "errors and omissions in documentation."

And in 2017, multiple patients suffered serious injuries at a rehabilitation center in Long Beach while under Telecare's supervision. The company said it would address the issues by randomly observing staff.

Telecare would not comment for this story.

When guests arrive at the Crowne Plaza, they receive a pamphlet instructing them to call Telecare if they're feeling "anxious, sad, or lonely," along with a list of phone numbers for emotional support and crisis response lines.

Together, Equus and Telecare can address any situation that may arise, said Nicole Ganier, vice president of operations for the western region of Equus.

"We recognize the complex nature of the population we serve as part of this program and have implemented policies and trained staff to assist them as effectively as possible," Ganier said in an email.

Addressing Emergencies

Teagle, the hotel site coordinator, said she loves her job, but Equus is overlooking opportunities to improve. The program is disorganized, staff aren't adequately trained, and guests who need help aren't getting it, she said.

She started working with Equus when the company was mass hiring in early December because of a COVID-19 outbreak at the San Diego Convention Center, where the city has an emergency homeless shelter. While she had experience working with people who are homeless, Teagle said she was unprepared for what she was thrown into at the Crowne Plaza.

As of February 12, about 300 people were isolating at the hotel.

Some are first responders and medical professionals who need to be isolated from their families because they've tested positive for the virus or have symptoms, but many are people without homes. Teagle said there are too many to adequately meet all of their needs.

The training Teagle said she received from Equus was minimal. She said the main message was: "Don't be a jerk."

There is no designated training coordinator, she said. Instead, workers are told to shadow each other, leading to inconsistent habits and procedures. Equus also doesn't explain to new staff exactly what Telecare's role is, other than that it provides resources for people in need.

Teagle said she was the first point of contact for many of the residents, yet nobody taught her how to look for signs of mental illness, drug addiction, or other issues that could come up. While staff are able to help with a range of problems, she said sometimes they just have to tell residents: "If you're feeling really bad, you've got to call 911."

San Diego police records show that after Equus and Telecare took over hotel operations for the county, calls from the Crowne Plaza continued to flood in.

Police have responded to more than 230 calls to the hotel since the pandemic began—three times more than the average number of calls seen in the prior two years. About a quarter of the calls were related to mental health, including suicide attempts and threats.

Summaries of the calls detailed 16 incidents where guests expressed suicidal thoughts. Some of the descriptions mentioned that residents were unhappy with staff or refused to leave the hotel after being discharged.

A San Diego police spokesperson confirmed two deaths have occurred at the hotel in the past two months, but details about those incidents are not yet available. A lieutenant who oversees patrols in the area declined to comment for this story.

"I Wasn't Breaking Any Rules"

Guests at the hotel are under a public health order, signed by county Public Health Officer Dr. Wilma Wooten, which requires them to isolate for at least 10 days. They aren't supposed to leave the hotel before then except for medical care.

But Teagle said that's not enforced. Security allows people to come and go, she said, and it's not uncommon for an entire day to pass before Equus realizes someone left early. She's also noticed the guards get in confrontations and "constantly have issues" with guests.

Two San Diegans who have stayed at the county's public health hotels told inewsource they have faced harassment from the security guards.

Morris, 60, lives with his wife, Martha, and his service dog, Mini-Me, in their gold Mitsubishi Outlander. He said they were offered a room in the Crowne Plaza after his wife tested positive for COVID-19 in November.

Within an hour, a security guard accosted him about leashing Mini-Me, who helps with his balance and mobility, he said.

Morris explained his dog doesn't wear a leash because he could trip over it, and the front desk already had the paperwork. The guard "rudely walked away," he said.

A document listing rules for guests at the hotel shows a leash isn't required if it impedes the service animal's ability to assist its owner.

Over nine days, Morris said the guards continued to berate him about the leash every time he went outside with Mini-Me.

"I don't know where they're getting these guys from. I don't know, are they pulling them off the street?" Morris said. "Because these guys are coming in... and doing a very good job of acting like thugs."

Equus signed a subcontract with AllState Security Services to run security at the Crowne Plaza. The San Diego-based agency's website says it provides private guards at construction sites, hospitals, schools, financial institutions and warehouses throughout California.

Ganier, the Equus representative, said all the companies they work with are vetted through background checks and pre-approved by the county. She wouldn't provide a full list of subcontractors or any details about their publicly funded work at the hotel, telling inewsource to ask the county for more information. The county did not provide a list of subcontractors either.

AllState didn't respond to requests for comment.

Morris said he reached his breaking point when a guard tried to hit him with a chair and two other guards intervened. Meanwhile, his wife was suffering from severe COVID-19 symptoms inside their room. Instead of focusing on her recovery, he said he was "busy fighting the wolves off."

He filed a complaint with Equus and left the hotel with more than a week remaining in his wife's stay. Equus and the county wouldn't comment on Morris's claims or any other allegations about the security guards.

He said he wished he could have stayed longer but feared one of the guards would try to hurt him.

"They were just on me every day, and every single day was a new situation with a new security guard, with a new issue of him proving himself that he was more of a man than I was, and I had to follow the rules," he said.

"The problem was, they had no idea I wasn't breaking any rules."

"These People Need Help"

As a site coordinator during the morning shift, Teagle said her responsibilities were to deliver breakfast and lunch, as well as tend to any other needs of those in isolation. That could mean coordinating a medical appointment or grocery pickups.

While caring for the residents, she said she started to notice a lack of empathy among Equus employees.

One day, she said a man who was formerly incarcerated called the front desk asking for an Android phone charger, saying the terms of his release required he keep his phone charged.

According to Teagle, her supervisor told her it didn't matter—the man could go to jail. She said she wound up finding a charger for him.

The problems she described went beyond empathy. Medications weren't distributed when they should have been, she said, causing some people to leave the hotel early. Medicine would sit in the hotel for days before workers delivered it to the guests, who were instructed not to leave their rooms because it could expose others to COVID-19.

Plus, nurses notified staff that toddlers at the hotel were losing weight because they weren't getting adequate nutrition, Teagle said. Equus planned to continue feeding toddlers milk or menu items such as quesadillas and lettuce wraps until she reached out to the food vendor to provide meals more appropriate for children—chicken and wild rice with sweet potatoes and applesauce, which are easier for toddlers to consume.

It was just a matter of communication, she said.

Teagle said she hasn't been to the Crowne Plaza since she was placed on leave earlier this month. She felt compelled to speak out because "these people need help."

"That could be my family," she said.

Cody Dulaney and Jill Castellano

Scathing SDSU Report Says County Contractors Were Unqualified to Operate COVID-19 Hotels

> *This story was originally produced and published by inewsource, a nonprofit, nonpartisan newsroom in San Diego committed to exposing wrongdoing and holding powerful people and institutions accountable. As part of their commitment to keeping the San Diego community informed, inewsource has allowed this story to be reprinted and shared here with you. To learn more about their work and how you can support their journalism, visit inewsource.org.*

August 4, 2021

San Diego County awarded a $30 million contract for operating COVID-19 hotels to an unqualified company with poorly trained staff, who forced residents to suffer through long delays for much-needed medication and who allowed for gaps in services that may have led to overdoses and suicide.

Those are among the findings outlined in a 154-page report released Tuesday from San Diego State University.

Why This Matters

San Diego County is spending millions of dollars to house people affected by COVID-19 in hotels. Some have tested positive or have symptoms, while others have health issues that put them at risk. Many are homeless and have no other place to safely isolate.

The school's Institute for Public Health evaluated the county's COVID-19 hotel sheltering program, which was meant to isolate people with the virus who had nowhere else to go.

The County Board of Supervisors ordered the review of the program in early March, eight days after an inewsource investigation uncovered poor care and oversight issues at the Crowne Plaza in Mission Valley—the main hotel used in the program.

Employees and hotel guests told SDSU that the county's contractor, Equus Workforce Solutions, is mismanaging the program, and staff aren't trained to work with many of those who are isolating—people who are homeless and might be struggling with mental illness or substance use disorders.

The report includes more than 40 confidential interviews with county employees, hotel program staff and guests. Most of the guests who responded to a survey had positive comments, but some describe harrowing experiences during SDSU interviews.

"Employees treat us like animals, without any compassion," a pregnant woman with two kids wrote in a complaint after leaving the program, according to the report.

"I don't want any family to go through what I went through. It's all inhumane," she added.

More key findings from the report include:

- Equus didn't have the credentials to operate this program, employed staff with no experience in social services, and didn't provide necessary training.
- The company responsible for mental health services, Telecare Corp., isn't equipped to meet guests' acute, complex, or severe mental health needs.
- Nurses and mental health specialists are not available 24 hours a day, even though guests are under a public health order to stay in their rooms while many suffer from COVID-19 symptoms.

- Some guests went hungry because they were repeatedly given meals they were allergic to or couldn't eat, and they were told their needs couldn't be met.

The county's contract with Equus is set to expire at the end of this year, but SDSU's report comes as COVID-19 cases surge across the region, and officials urge the public to take more precautions.

The county agreed in April to pay SDSU $140,000 to review the strengths and weaknesses of the COVID-19 hotels, as well as offer recommendations.

County spokesperson Michael Workman defended the sheltering program, saying it "stood up in response to an unprecedented pandemic."

"This Public Health program was designed to mitigate community spread of COVID-19 among residents who needed isolation shelter," Workman said. "Either because they had tested positive or were in a high-risk environment. It was not intended to be a shelter or a hospital."

The county's full response:

> The COVID-19 Emergency Non-Congregate Shelter Program was stood up in response to an unprecedented pandemic. This Public Health program was designed to mitigate community spread of COVID-19 among residents who needed isolation shelter. Either because they had tested positive or were in a high-risk environment. It was not intended to be a shelter or a hospital.
>
> The County and our contracted service providers have been extremely responsive to the evolving needs of this program, including implementing programmatic changes to improve services throughout the duration of the response. To illustrate the changing nature of the program, the clients populating most of our rooms now are asylum seekers waiting out isolation or quarantine.

The evaluation of the program is indicative of the County Board of Supervisors' commitment to continual improvement of our services.

It is equally important to note the critical successes of this program:

- 100% success in preventing COVID-19 outbreaks within the program
- 93% success rate in guests staying for the recommended length of time
- High percentage of positive guest satisfaction surveys

We look forward to working with our partners, contracted and otherwise, to strengthen our response to health and other emergencies now and in the future, and this report will be taken into account in those next steps.

Michael Workman
Director, County Communications Office

Nathan Fletcher, chair of the county board of supervisors, could not be reached for comment by publication time.

The final report commends county and contract employees for their dedication to the program, for moving quickly to get the program started, and for adapting under constantly changing circumstances. It lists 10 strengths, including that the vast majority of people completed their isolation and quarantine period. The program likely prevented the spread of COVID-19 across the county, SDSU said.

But the review also confirms much of inewsource's previous reporting about poor care and gaps in services for people in isolation. The SDSU authors found that no county employee is responsible for overseeing all aspects of the program, and they couldn't determine if anyone has ultimate decision-making authority.

"Staff at all levels report confusion about who is responsible for various aspects of the program," the report said. "Clear answers about program operations and program data were difficult for the evaluation team to obtain."

SDSU offered nine recommendations to improve the program, one of which included 14 changes that could be made right away to address concerns raised by staff and guests. They include staffing nurses and mental health specialists around the clock, ensuring medications are delivered on time, and assessing guests for mental health needs when they arrive at the hotel.

Unqualified

In March 2020, San Diego County started using the Crowne Plaza and other hotels to house people who had nowhere else to isolate from the coronavirus. That included first responders who needed to be away from family as well as people without housing.

The stated goal of the hotel sheltering program was twofold: to isolate people who test positive or come in contact with the virus and to protect people who are at-risk for developing severe illness. In a six-month period, the program served more than 5,500 people.

The at-risk hotels are available to people who are medically compromised or experiencing homelessness, and while they were not included in the report, SDSU recommended they be evaluated as well.

SDSU found that the program was up and running within a week, and to keep it operating, county employees continue to make many personal and professional sacrifices. But the program has been plagued with problems from the start.

In an email inewsource obtained last spring, one county employee told colleagues she was "pushing and begging and pleading for additional staff" to help provide adequate support.

Within a week, county officials changed an existing $13 million contract it had with Telecare, which had been providing mental health services to San Diegans in the legal system, to also help people in isolation.

But multiple people told SDSU that Telecare wasn't equipped to work with people isolating in the hotels.

"Telecare is behavioral health lite," one county employee said. "It is not for acute care. It can't be used for crisis stabilization."

Not long after Telecare became involved, 28-year-old Jose Angel Gomez-Camacho died by suicide at the Crowne Plaza. The death wasn't discovered for five days.

Telecare would not comment for this story.

Gomez-Camacho's autopsy report said he had checked out of the hotel but was somehow able to gain reentry before his death. The SDSU review explains that keeping track of guests has been a recurring problem for the program: Staff have trouble tracking who's supposed to arrive at the hotel, where they're coming from, and who has already checked in.

Two months after inewsource uncovered the suicide death, county officials hired Equus to take over the hotel sheltering program.

The report found Equus was able to provide lodging services within one month. But that was the staffing agency's main focus. Equus wasn't prepared to handle other parts of the job, such as working with homeless and mentally ill people.

Hiring Equus was like fitting "a square peg in a round hole," one employee said.

An Equus representative did not respond to a request for comment.

Multiple people told SDSU that any contractor running the program needed to have extensive experience offering around-the-clock care, with "a team of medical folks, mental health experts, and residential experts in place," the report said.

But county staff members disagreed about the type of program that was needed. Some said the goal was simply to house people and reduce community spread, while others recognized it would become a shelter serving primarily vulnerable people with complex needs.

"Equus had good intentions, but they were not prepared to do behavioral health or social services work," one person told SDSU.

A lack of experience and training among Equus staff played a big role, the report found.

Equus's medical director had no experience in infectious disease or public health, the report said, and was hired because of his background administering over-the-counter medications.

Each Equus employee interviewed by SDSU said they had only received on-the-job training and a large binder of operating procedures they were expected to review on their own. No one received formal training on behavioral health, trauma-informed care, or de-escalation techniques. One staff member said the person in Human Resources who hired him couldn't even describe the job duties. Frontline employees weren't given the tools to help those in need.

"I have no background or training in social support. My manager told me my experience with multitasking would be enough," one Equus employee said.

Gaps in Care

According to their contracts with the county, Equus and Telecare are supposed to provide case management and wraparound services to meet people's unique needs. That covers everything from cash assistance and housing navigation to mental health and substance use disorders.

SDSU found some case management has happened. The majority of people experiencing homelessness before entering the program returned to another shelter setting, while 22 people moved into permanent supportive housing, which was considered "an impressive accomplishment," the report said.

But no single person is assigned to a guest to oversee all aspects of their care. Instead, the services are provided piecemeal, and responsibilities are divided among multiple staff members.

"These gaps in care coordination may have led to both overdoses and suicide," one county staff member said.

Employees also had difficulty managing guests with substance use disorders. County staff acknowledged that drug activity has been a concern, and one guest described "rampant drug use" and drugs being smuggled in through food delivery bags that went unsearched.

"This is a terrible place if you are in recovery—there are people actively using all around you," a county staff member said.

SDSU recommended investigating whether it is possible to limit deliveries and start searching belongings.

Calls to San Diego police about problems at these hotels have continued flooding in ever since the program started, records show. About 1 in 10 of the calls were related to mental health, including suicide attempts and threats, according to a recent analysis.

But even when violence, drug use, and suicide attempts occur in the hotels, San Diego police are reluctant to intervene, the report said.

Once a person has keys to a hotel room, according to county staff, it is then considered their property and police can only enter under extreme circumstances.

One employee described a traumatic experience with a guest experiencing suicidal ideation and psychosis, where law enforcement refused to do anything unless staff observed an attempt being made.

"They are following the rule book," a county employee said of San Diego police, "but the rule book doesn't work in a crisis like this."

"They're Trying to Fix It"

The SDSU review corroborated stories from employees and guests who have exposed neglect and wrongdoing in the sheltering program in inewsource reporting over the past year and a half.

A former Equus employee, Turquoise Teagle, in interviews with inewsource criticized the county for not closely monitoring the program on site, instead relying on daily video calls with staff. She also described guests waiting days for medication and not receiving adequate food—all of which have been supported by the new report.

"I had diarrhea and was vomiting, but I had to wait for medication," one guest told SDSU. Another said he started feeling sick after the program's nurse left work and couldn't get help until the next day.

"I thought it would be more intense medical care because we had COVID," someone else in the program said. "I was worried I was going to die. If I had a choice, I would have stayed home where I felt safer."

According to the report, many guests complained they were hungry, food portion sizes were too small, staff wouldn't provide snacks, and they limited the amount of water each person could have. One person said they were repeatedly given meat even though they don't have molars. Another said they were provided ham sandwiches even though they don't eat pork.

SDSU's review brought up another frequently cited issue among those in the sheltering program—AllState Security guards.

While some guests said they had no issues with security, others recounted waking up to the sounds of guards screaming in the middle of the night. One heard a guard yelling at a guest that they "need to shut up and get in [their] room," and another witnessed a violent altercation between two guards.

Equus acknowledged that ensuring adequate, respectful security has been problematic, the report says.

A representative with AllState Security Service did not respond to an interview request.

William Morris, who went to the Crowne Plaza last November after his wife tested positive for COVID-19, said he has faced harassment and physical violence from security guards. A dispute about his service dog escalated to a guard attempting to hit him with a chair, he told inewsource in February. Records show he also reported the incident to Equus.

But ever since inewsource reported these issues earlier this year, he said his experience in the program has greatly improved.

"Thank God somebody, somewhere started talking, having meetings, and it's a lot better. It really is," Morris said in an interview last week.

Morris was living in a gold Mitsubishi Outlander with his wife and 11-year-old Havanese service dog named Mini-Me. But they've been staying in one of the at-risk hotels managed by Equus in Old Town since January.

"It got out of hand, and now they're trying to fix it," Morris said, later adding that "these people are doing a wonderful job.

"You have a lot of people who care," he added, "and you can see it the way they speak to people, you can see it the way they look at people, you can see it the way they walk away from people."

Moving forward, SDSU recommended that the county increase oversight of future programs, contract with qualified service providers with extensive experience, and focus on medical and behavioral health services.

County officials have not announced when the report will be reviewed at a public board meeting or what it will mean for the future of services provided at the hotels.

Workman, the county spokesperson, said SDSU's review shows the county's commitment to continually improving its services. He added that the county has worked with its contractors to adapt to quickly changing situations over the course of the pandemic.

"We look forward to working with our partners, contracted and otherwise, to strengthen our response to health and other emergencies now and in the future," Workman said, "and this report will be taken into account in those next steps."

refugees

Roxana Popescu

Pandemic Blew Open Digital Equity Chasm for San Diego's Refugees. What's Next?

> *This story was originally produced and published by inewsource, a nonprofit, nonpartisan newsroom in San Diego committed to exposing wrongdoing and holding powerful people and institutions accountable. As part of their commitment to keeping the San Diego community informed, inewsource has allowed this story to be reprinted and shared here with you. To learn more about their work and how you can support their journalism, visit inewsource.org.*

May 24, 2021

Growing up in Syria, Douha Alhalabi rarely had to use a computer, let alone Google. Back then and there, things were handled "in paper."

Today her home is El Cajon, where she's been trying to find work, attend college, apply for rental assistance—all online. It's left her deeply frustrated.

When someone sent her to a "www dot" internet address, she didn't know what "dot" meant and didn't find the web page. When she tried to Google something, she didn't know what exactly to type.

"It does damage my family, yes, because we have no idea how to use technology," she said.

As with the thousands of other refugees who live in San Diego County, that "damage" has reverberated across Alhalabi's life this past year during the COVID-19 pandemic.

She and her husband haven't been able to work remotely. Telehealth appointments became impossible without a translator. Online unemployment and rental assistance applications were so daunting, she gave up figuring them out on her own. The family became vulnerable to exploitation by "professional" people, as Alhalabi called them—third parties who helped them fill out those "hard applications" for hefty fees.

Now, as vaccination rates rise and in-person schools and businesses reopen, many experiences that shifted online may stay that way. That puts some of the region's refugees at risk of being shut out of the economic recovery, because they lack the digital skills and adequate internet access that are as essential to life in San Diego as understanding traffic rules and being proficient in English.

That digital inequity has also contributed to deep job losses in San Diego's refugee communities. According to one nonprofit, the unemployment rate in the fall of 2020 among refugees was more than three times higher than the county average at that time: 22% versus 6.6%.

What's next for those families? Perhaps eviction, perhaps not finding new jobs because of big gaps in their resumes, said Homayra Yusufi, the interim executive director of Partnership for the Advancement of New Americans, a local community organizing, research and public policy nonprofit.

"I think it's going to definitely play out worse for those folks who have digital inequities," she said.

These gaps could soon impact even more refugees in San Diego County. This month, President Joe Biden raised the limit on how many refugees the U.S. admits, more than quadrupling this year's cap set by the Trump administration, from 15,000 to 62,500.

Community organizations say they are trying to help refugees by teaching digital literacy classes, donating computers, translating websites, and converting their employees into internet navigation mentors.

Yusufi said her nonprofit and other groups are offering a "kind of patchwork relief, wherever we can." That, she added, is because instead of making "real investments and foresight," governments at all levels are underinvesting in refugee services. Nonprofits receive varying amounts of government funding to pay for some refugee programs but not enough to support the needs of all the people they serve.

"The fact that we rely on nonprofits to be providing basic services to the entire population, I think there's always going to be holes there, because we know nonprofits are also financially struggling," Yusufi said. "There'll always be issues like that unless we can make that investment—unless the government, be it local, county, state, federal, can prioritize those things and actually put the budget behind it to address those issues."

As Ramah Awad, a community organizer with Majdal: The Arab Community Center of San Diego, sees it, nonprofits are filling gaps that the county government should be filling in its role to provide social services that improve the socioeconomic circumstances of those in need.

"Instead of it being embedded and integrated into the county's infrastructure, it's being outsourced to different nonprofits," she said. "So I think there is a tension there. Who should be doing this work, and is it sustainable?"

Such work is critical, she added, because families' long-term stability hinges upon it.

Her conclusion: "If their access to applying to jobs, their access to classes for English language, if all of that is predicated on knowing how to fill out online forms, create online accounts, accessing a laptop—if all of that is predicated on digital access, then I think that it really is a stepping stone to being able to access all the other services that can get them to better socioeconomic standing in the longer term."

Basic Digital Needs Unmet

In the old days, before the pandemic, Abraham Tessema used to drive people to medical appointments and help them fill out applications.

"Most of them are farmers. They've never been in educational settings," he said of the Etheopian and Eritrean families he works with at the Refugee Assistance Center in City Heights. "That's been a challenge—to even open a letter and read it and understand what it is saying. So they would bring it to us."

During the pandemic his roles have been sharpened and focused into one: translating the internet. "The problem here is they cannot do the basic steps," he said. "The language barrier comes first. They don't even understand what to do."

Etleva Bejko, the director of Refugee and Immigration Services with Jewish Family Service of San Diego, a refugee resettlement agency, realized early in the pandemic that new immigrants must understand the internet in order to get updates about the fast-changing situation.

"Imagine being new in a country, not understanding the language, and on top of that a worldwide pandemic is happening," Bejko said. "Digital literacy has become as important, if not more important, than any of the other topics that we require and teach in our cultural orientation."

The agency joined a pilot program developed by its parent nonprofit, HIAS, where mentors who speak Ukrainian, Farsi, or Pashto teach refugees how to use a computer for online banking, telehealth, technical skills and, in parallel, English.

Bejko said of one refugee: "When she started the pilot, she didn't even know how to turn the device on. And now she's independently using it." The local program has 10 participants and will continue for five more months. So far, she said, participants' reactions have been "very positive."

For every refugee who gets help and training, hundreds don't, service providers said.

"We're just not able to get to all of them," said Awad, with the Majdal Center, adding that she and a part-time worker help two to three families a week with digital access issues. About 250 families on their roster could use help, she said.

Tessema said his organization is helping 36 families, while 200 "desperately" need support. "This is in our eyes the people that we can see," he added. "And there are other refugee groups, like the Congolese, the Rwandans. I see that they needed help. We haven't even touched that part yet."

"It's Not for Us"

Digital literacy and access are, on one hand, a "bottleneck," Tessema said. Without them, people can't access resources, jobs, or information. On the other hand, for refugees specifically, digital equity is also tangled with other challenges: language, cultural differences, fragile finances, and unfamiliarity with systems and norms in the U.S.

When the pandemic pushed many of her interactions online, Alaa Taha, 28, a refugee from Syria, didn't trust telemedicine. That, combined with her low confidence in her English abilities, led her to opt out of doctor appointments. She's also felt overwhelmed by her two kids' remote classes and her own college coursework in business administration.

Twice since the pandemic began, she needed a doctor's care for an acute health problem. Instead, she canceled both visits.

"It's not normal to talk with the doctor online and explain the pain, how do you feel, to the doctor. It should [be] the doctor sees the patient," Taha said.

Dilkhwaz Ahmed, the executive director of License to Freedom, an El Cajon nonprofit that's been helping Taha, has also seen people give up on vital economic support because they felt overwhelmed by requirements and unfamiliar, complex websites and software.

"By the end, they say, you know what? Forget about it. It's not for us," Ahmed said.

She recalled a man who joked that a rental assistance application had to be for a job with the U.S. State Department because it was so complicated.

"This link, it's designed for American people who know the language, and they know how to access the internet, so they can fill it out and they can upload," he told her. Then, he added, "You know what? This is not for me. This program is not designed for me." He did not apply at the time, she added.

These scenarios point to the complexity of teaching and helping refugees and other immigrants navigate the digital chasms that have been torn open during the pandemic. Their problems go beyond slow internet, or not enough devices, or not understanding how to use Zoom. It's all of those compounded by limited language ability and overlapping layers of unfamiliarity with digital tools and with how things work in the U.S.

Shatha Dahash, once a lawyer in Iraq and now the case manager helping Taha, said language, technical competence, and trust in systems go hand in hand.

When one is missing, Dahash said, "Everything will be hard."

More dire than health, even in a pandemic, are family finances, service providers said. Without digital literacy and access to computers or adequate internet connections for remote work, many refugees have had trouble holding on to jobs or applying for new jobs. And for those who have lost work, the same tech barriers make it hard to apply for unemployment, food stamps, or rental assistance.

Yusufi, with the Partnership for the Advancement of New Americans in City Heights, said digital inequity will be less of a problem with schools reopening and things like in-person doctor visits picking up. But she's wary of expecting things to go back to "normal." In the post-pandemic economy, some jobs aren't coming back, and others will stay remote, she said.

"I think that the bigger issue for our communities is also what does that mean, particularly for their incomes, particularly for employment opportunities and being able to have enough to sustain a family," she said.

The results so far are not encouraging for refugees, service providers said. When industries that typically employed refugees, such as hospitality, transportation, childcare and food service, let workers go last year because of stay-at-home orders, an instant impact of the digital gap was economic. Unable to work in person or remotely, refugees lost jobs.

A forthcoming report by Yusufi's nonprofit, based on a survey last fall of 544 of the region's refugees, says 22% were unemployed and looking for work, and 51% were not looking for work because they were students or had given up job hunting.

"The biggest challenge of all is access to employment opportunities," Bejko agreed. That's not just the case for refugees, she added, but they tend to be isolated and not have the local context, experience, or contacts that others might.

Even with support from nonprofits, the impact on refugees, including Alhalabi and her family, who are adjusting to a new way of life in El Cajon, both offline and online, has been devastating. She and her husband lost work during the pandemic, and she said they wanted to find jobs.

She was a childcare provider, and her husband was an Uber driver, two hard-hit industries.

Because she couldn't figure out the internet, Alhalabi missed a federal financial aid application that would have funded her ESL classes, positioning her for better work opportunities, and she said her daughter missed a college application deadline, leading to a "lost" year.

To apply for rental assistance, food stamps, unemployment, and college financial aid, the family paid around $700 to a third party to help them.

Ahmed said these "fixers" are exploiting refugees. "People are asking them to pay $100 in order to help them with the applications. It's terrible," she said. "People just try to take advantage of those people who don't speak English by applying for them."

Whose Problem?

With refugees needing digital help, some community organizations said they've been forced to shift their focus.

Tessema said the Refugee Assistance Center had to "jump into this."

The Majdal Center, whose mission is to "uplift" its community members through advocacy and cultural programming, is now doing tech support to help people with online rental assistance applications.

"We, as a center, are not built to do the social service work…but because of the pandemic we had to pivot," Awad said. "And so we're making do with what resources we have."

Several local refugee groups applied to the state for a grant to combat health and digital inequity, but it was recently denied.

Bejko, with Jewish Family Service, said nonprofits step in to provide services until broader solutions from others emerge. "As everybody figures it out, what's the best way to conduct business, the need is still there. So we do have to help our clients, even though that adds to the list of items, of services or gaps or challenges we have to help remove," she said.

Yusufi said she wished government agencies had done more. State lawmakers responded with Senate Bill 91, which extends eviction protection through June, and the San Diego Unified School District equipped students with internet hotspots.

To prevent refugees from ending up "worse off" as the pandemic wanes, she said her nonprofit advocates for "bold policy changes," not "short-term relief programs."

She is thinking big: reconsidering the resettlement system, helping refugees find affordable housing so they're not living in overcrowded conditions. These ideas extend beyond digital equity, but she said they get at the same goal: investing in refugees for their long-term success.

Bejko said the goal for refugees going through resettlement is "self-sufficiency." The pilot program—the one that teaches everything from online banking to English—is one step in that direction. Another is emphasizing the internet is "a necessity," she said, instead of something merely "good to have."

Like electricity, gas, and water, she added.

Along with being guided by nonprofits, some refugees are learning new digital literacy skills on their own.

Alhalabi said she has been watching YouTube videos to learn about "technology stuff," and asks her kids and husband to explain things to her.

Taha, in her El Cajon apartment, her two young sons giggling in the next room, said she feels she has been getting more competent with each online adventure.

"It's still hard, but I learn," she said, then opened her laptop to get some work done.

Roxana Popescu
Pandemic Takes a Toll on San Diego County Refugees Sheltering in Place With Abusive Partners

> *This story was originally produced and published by inewsource, a nonprofit, nonpartisan newsroom in San Diego committed to exposing wrongdoing and holding powerful people and institutions accountable. As part of their commitment to keeping the San Diego community informed, inewsource has allowed this story to be reprinted and shared here with you. To learn more about their work and how you can support their journalism, visit inewsource.org.*

June 9, 2020

A 31-year-old woman was hiding in the laundry room of her El Cajon apartment building. She needed help.

Her husband, 41, lost his job during the COVID-19 pandemic and was taking out his anger on her. She called Dilkhwaz Ahmed, who works with refugee victims of domestic violence.

"It's harder now because he's at home all the time," the woman said.

The pandemic has taken a toll on women who are sheltering in place with abusive partners.

For some refugees and immigrants, like this woman, the situation is even more fraught. They can be isolated and don't always speak English well. Many don't understand the legal system and local resources. And some fear getting help or leaving an abusive partner could jeopardize their ability to stay in the U.S.

"Our refugee and immigrant community is already one of the most vulnerable populations, even in the best of times, because they experience unique challenges," said Stephanie Baez, a supervising attorney with the San Diego Volunteer Lawyer Program. "Right now, during this pandemic, those issues are magnified."

Since San Diego County's COVID-19 health restrictions took effect in March, the El Cajon nonprofit that Ahmed heads, License to Freedom, has seen an uptick in calls for help. Victims have tended to reach out when their situations are more dire, she added.

Ahmed said that in some cases abusers have used religion and immigration status to isolate and terrorize victims—for example, saying the pandemic is an opportunity to reconcile and that God will punish them if they do not cooperate. Or, she said, they threaten to send their wives back to their countries. Women also get pressured by members of their communities to stay married, she added.

The pandemic and the self-isolation that came with it have created a situation where women are stuck in close quarters with their abusers, making it hard for them to step outside, get a break, and seek help, local experts said. And if they do get out and make a call, social distancing guidelines have made shelter beds more scarce, and both shelter beds and unofficial channels—a friend's or relative's couch—are less available as people keep apart to stay healthy.

El Cajon police and the Sheriff's Department, which patrols a significant part of East County, both report increases in domestic violence–related incidents during the first two months of the coronavirus shutdowns.

Though the agencies don't record if the incidents involved refugees, it's well known that many refugees have settled in East County. More than 24,000 people born in Iraq lived in San Diego County in 2018, and more than half of them lived in El Cajon, according to census data. About 3,400 Syrians live in San Diego County, as well.

"I Need to Get Out Now"

Ahmed estimated her workload has shifted from about 70% domestic violence crisis intervention before the pandemic to 90% now. In March, April, and May, she had 15 new cases each month—up from 10 in February.

"We are at court every day filing restraining orders, almost," Ahmed said.

The reports surfacing are also more extreme, said Claudia Grasso, assistant chief of the Family Protection Division of the District Attorney's Office.

"Our hotline providers, they're saying that they're not necessarily getting an uptick in calls, but the calls that they are getting are more urgent. Basically, 'I need to get out now' type of calls," Grasso said. She wants victims to know that services are still available, even if in some cases they are remote for now.

Ahmed's office got one such frantic call in April from a woman whose husband had threatened her with his gun. The 42-year-old woman said her husband verbally degraded her and their children when they asked what he did with the family's stimulus money, issued by the federal government to offset income losses caused by the pandemic.

The man, a security guard, grabbed his gun and threatened his wife and children. The next day, the wife filed a restraining order.

"I'm very scared for my kids and for my life," she told inewsource.

She was one of eight domestic violence victims inewsource interviewed for this story. Because the women fear for their safety, inewsource agreed to not publish their names.

Across the country from mid-March to early May, about 5,600 people reached out to the National Domestic Violence Hotline and mentioned the COVID-19 pandemic, or about a tenth of all contacts.

"COVID-19 is being used by abusive partners to further control and abuse," said Christina So, communications director of the National Domestic Violence Hotline.

Calls for help didn't initially increase when the pandemic hit, but that has been changing as stay-home orders begin to loosen. "Survivors have been in close proximity to their abusers, and it may have been less safe to reach out for support," So said in an email. A "small increase" in calls for help is starting as stay-at-home orders are scaled back, she added.

In El Cajon, police reported domestic abuse–related calls increased 14% in March and April compared to the same period last year, going from 362 to 413.

For the parts of East County served by the Sheriff's Department, including Santee, Lemon Grove, and Rancho San Diego, domestic violence–related calls and deputy actions increased 4% in March and April compared to the same months in 2019.

Baez, the lawyer, said domestic abusive behavior doesn't look different across cultures—it is about "control"—but refugee victims might have "cultural or religious beliefs that make it harder to break free from an abusive relationship." Some households might also be on shakier financial ground but not be entitled to the same benefits as U.S. citizens, adding to tensions, she said. Most crucial: refugees' isolation.

"The biggest issue is just not knowing how to seek help and not having anywhere to go," Baez said.

Refugees Need to Know Help Is Available

Domestic abuse hotlines have English and Spanish speakers but typically not speakers fluent in Arabic, Farsi, or Chaldean, said Grasso with the District Attorney's Office. The hotlines can bring in a third-party translator—but things get lost in translation.

"It's tough when you're not bicultural, when you don't understand the culture, and you're trying to assist that victim. I mean, there is that added layer of difficulty," Grasso said.

During the pandemic, Ahmed added, it's even harder for victims of abuse to find temporary housing with a friend or family member, as people have limited in-person contacts to avoid infection.

Most of Ahmed's crisis intervention work is done by phone today, in Arabic. Victims open up about their troubles online and get Ahmed's contact info through the Viber app, which some in San Diego's refugee communities have been using to stay in touch during the pandemic. Then they call her—or, in one case, a victim's mother reached out to Ahmed from Iraq on behalf of her daughter in El Cajon.

Once she connects with victims, Ahmed often has to educate them about things like restraining orders and their rights. In one case, she convinced a woman to get a restraining order against her husband despite the woman's fear of angering him. As she hesitated, he filed one against his wife and took their two children.

The woman, from Syria, told inewsource that her husband has "anger issues" and was violent.

"He doesn't have patience," she said. "When the kids ask for something, he will hit. And when he hits, he hits so hard." She has since met with an attorney.

Ahmed said she alerted county Child Welfare Services about her situation, but the children weren't removed from the father.

"Please, please help me to see my kids. I want them," the woman told inewsource.

Asked about the woman's claim, a county spokeswoman described in a statement how Child Welfare Services responds to reports of child abuse. After a report is made, a screener uses a decision-making tool to determine if the report "meets the threshold for investigation."

"If there are concerns regarding an investigation, CWS recommends first contacting the [Protective Services Worker] and their supervisor to discuss the situation. If the complaint cannot be resolved at that level, CWS has an Office of the Ombudsman that conducts independent reviews of complaints concerning policies or practices," she said.

Ahmed did coax another woman to file a restraining order in April. The wife and her husband argued about whether to follow the shelter-in-place restrictions. He threw food at her—the breakfast she'd cooked for him, his favorite kind of eggs, the wife said. Then he pushed her to the ground, grabbed her by the legs and hit her in the face, she said. She sought treatment from a doctor.

When the sobbing woman made excuses for her husband, saying his mother was the problem, Ahmed told her in a recent phone call: "You don't want [your child] to grow up seeing you being hit by her dad."

The woman is pregnant with the couple's second child, and their first is a year old. She hopes her husband will behave better. She is anxious about her future.

"I try to be fine," she said.

With stay-at-home orders being eased, domestic violence experts are uncertain about what it might mean for women living in abusive situations.

The National Domestic Violence Hotline expects to see an unprecedented number of calls for help in the coming months.

And whichever way the trends go as society reopens, Grasso said she hopes domestic violence victims get help.

Create a Domestic Violence Safety Plan

Claudio Grasso is the assistant chief of the Family Protection Division of the District Attorney's Office and president of the San Diego Domestic Violence Council, which works to prevent and reduce these crimes.

Grasso shared pointers on how to put together a domestic violence safety plan.

- Identify an area of the house where there are no weapons. If things start getting volatile with your partner, go to that place.
- If you're being chased, don't run to where the children are, to protect them.
- Have a phone with you at all times.
- Have a code word with trusted neighbors or friends. If you say this code word, they understand that they are to call the police immediately.
- Teach your kids to call 911. Have a code word with the children.
- Have a bag packed with clothes, essentials, and cash. Put it in the trunk of your car.
- Park your car so it's easy to get in and out. (For example, don't park so you'd have to back out. That would be more difficult.)
- Particularly important: Try not to wear scarves or jewelry or anything that can be used to strangle.

Roxana Popescu

"It's Do or Die For Them." Life for San Diego's Refugees Was Tough. Then Came COVID-19.

> *This story was originally produced and published by inewsource, a nonprofit, nonpartisan newsroom in San Diego committed to exposing wrongdoing and holding powerful people and institutions accountable. As part of their commitment to keeping the San Diego community informed, inewsource has allowed this story to be reprinted and shared here with you. To learn more about their work and how you can support their journalism, visit inewsource.org.*

October 15, 2020

San Diego's Karen refugees, an ethnic minority of Burma, are used to uncertainty.

They were persecuted, their villages burned. They fled through jungles, not knowing if they would meet life or death. The survivors waited for decades in refugee camps for permission to start over somewhere new.

That's why for the Karen people and for other refugees and asylum seekers from around the world who have resettled in San Diego, COVID-19 has been one more blow, said Nao Kabashima, executive director of the nonprofit Karen Organization of San Diego.

The pandemic has left them unemployed, reluctant to seek medical care, and at risk for eviction. The children of these refugees, like many others, aren't adjusting well to online education, but their parents are less equipped than others to guide them.

Some of these challenges will be long lasting, Kabashima fears.

"I am afraid that it would take a long time for many refugees to get jobs again," she said. "I think about that every day."

Until recently, many of these concerns were anecdotal. But a first-of-its-kind survey, released Thursday by the San Diego Refugee Communities Coalition, concretely details how deeply the pandemic has impacted immigrants and refugees from across the region—from healthcare to education to imperiled basic needs such as housing, food, and physical safety.

Amina Sheik Mohamed, the director of the Refugee Health Unit with the University of California San Diego's Center for Community Health, and one of the survey's facilitators, said it was carried out in a unique way.

"This is different," Sheik Mohamed said. "It's very much engaged with the community.... It was not like a typical researcher coming and doing research to the community, but it was really co-designed. The community leaders are conducting it."

The communities tapped their own members to conduct extensive phone and in-person interviews in 12 languages about the pandemic's impact on 306 families, granting the researchers unprecedented access to people who might otherwise not have been listened to. Because of that, Sheik Mohamed said, the findings reach across communities to learn about problems and gaps in services that have affected thousands of immigrants from different backgrounds.

The survey found that during the pandemic:

- Almost a third of families canceled or missed health appointments.
- In more than 40% of families, at least one member lost a job or was laid off.
- 60% of families couldn't pay all of their rent.

- Over a third of families said they are afraid they'll be evicted. More recent immigrants and families with bigger households are at greater risk.

The family members interviewed were from countries including Afghanistan, Burma, the Democratic Republic of the Congo, Haiti, Somalia, Sudan, and Syria. Because the survey asked about their entire households, researchers learned about the situations of more than 1,400 people.

Some problems were acute.

"I was paying rent up until now, but now I can't since the rental assistance program is over. I do not know what I can do," one person told an interviewer. Another said, "I need help with rent. PLEASE."

A concern underlying the survey's findings is refugees will have a hard time bouncing back after the pandemic.

"Families with school-age children are concerned about the impact that school closures and changes to how education is delivered will have a long-term impact on learning," the report said. "Community leaders are concerned that inequities that existed pre-COVID-19 will be exacerbated."

The report also identified areas where needs are being met within the communities themselves or by public programs and nonprofits. But it also found gaps between the support and resources being offered and what is needed and proposed solutions.

Kabashima, who coordinated the survey and outreach for Karen and other refugees from Burma, said the results were concerning but not surprising, revealing how widespread problems are.

The survey, she said, confirmed that all of the region's refugee communities are suffering and struggling with the same issues as the Karen people.

"It was also shocking to know how many families actually are struggling from unemployment," she added.

A Grassroots Survey

One reason the survey is unusual is that it was designed and carried out by a grassroots group of ethnic community-based organizations that make up the San Diego Refugee Communities Coalition.

This survey is the first time that these discrete refugee ethnic organizations and nonprofits have come together to examine from the grassroots the circumstances and concerns around the impact of the coronavirus pandemic on their communities.

Valerie Nash, a consultant who helped develop the survey's report, said that in the past City Heights, a diverse mid-city neighborhood where many of San Diego's refugees live, has been studied and examined extensively but typically by outside entities.

She said the grassroots nature of this survey, with people interviewing members of their own communities, meant refugees could identify and investigate the issues they deemed important.

Rebecca Fielding-Miller, an assistant professor of infectious disease and global public health at UCSD, said this kind of research helps ensure that the response to the pandemic protects society's more vulnerable members, which in turn helps everybody.

"None of us are safe until the people at the highest risk are safe. It's an airborne infectious disease. To me, as a public health social scientist, the thing that we always need to be building for is ensuring that the people at the margins are taken care of," Fielding-Miller said. "Because when they're taken care of, everybody is taken care of."

Research, she added, can also shape policy.

"Policy responds to data, right?" Fielding-Miller said.

In this case, she said, being able to "translate a known, lived experience amongst a marginalized community" to something that can be demonstrated and measured is key because it helps create policy and direct where money should go to help these refugees.

The report states its goal is to understand the pandemic's impact on refugees, inform solutions, and "mobilize action." It concludes with dozens of recommendations for addressing those needs and gaps in services.

For education, improving parents' digital literacy and providing more tech support to families would help children better adjust to online schooling.

For healthcare, one of the long-term recommendations is investment in "culturally responsive services and treatment," while under housing, a short-term solution the report identified is to extend rental relief programs past October, the report said.

Deep Economic Pain

Meshate Mengistu, the community health coordinator at United Women of East Africa, one of 11 San Diego refugee groups that helped conduct the survey, said the families she spoke with in August and September were struggling to afford basic needs.

"Do they feed their children [or] decide whether they buy diapers for their young children?" she said.

The pandemic has exacerbated the financial difficulties of refugees, who already were more likely to struggle to meet basic needs, the survey noted.

"Our community members were working in the very industries which were hard hit by this: the restaurant industry, hotel industry, and tourism industry," said Kabashima with the Karen nonprofit.

Among those who answered questions about income and employment, about a quarter said they worked fewer hours, more than 40% lost jobs or were laid off, and others were expecting to lose a job. Twelve people said their families had to close businesses because of the pandemic.

These findings, compared with the high unemployment figures for areas of the county where refugees and immigrants tend to live, are another window into how low-income and immigrant communities have disproportionately borne the brunt of the pandemic's economic devastation.

Some of the families surveyed estimated their income shortly before and during the pandemic—in January and July. Almost three-quarters of them lost income, with an average decrease of 29%, or $846 a month.

The survey also found that 23% of all the families interviewed were "extremely concerned" about being able to afford food, and almost all received some kind of assistance, including an economic stimulus check, Pandemic EBT—one-time funding to cover children's meals—or unemployment.

Education and Health Gaps

For refugees new to the U.S. who are trying to figure out unfamiliar school and health systems, the pandemic has made adjusting harder.

Access to healthcare is complex, with more than half of the people surveyed saying they prefer in-person medical visits over video and phone consultations. About a third said they have skipped or canceled medical appointments because they were afraid of contracting COVID-19, didn't have childcare, were concerned about privacy and language barriers, or were quarantining with coronavirus symptoms.

More than 50,000 people in San Diego County have tested positive for the coronavirus. It's not known how many were refugees, but COVID-19 case counts have been higher in ZIP codes where those who took the survey live, including El Cajon, the College Area, and City Heights.

The pandemic has "really amplified and magnified things that we know were already happening," Fielding-Miller with UCSD said. "Those issues are now happening through the lens of COVID, and they are even more obvious than they were."

She said even when refugees and immigrants "do have access to insurance, we know that finding a provider who is culturally competent is difficult."

"We know that getting care from a provider that is on par with what essentially an affluent White peer would get is difficult because systemic racism is inherent in the medical system," Fielding-Miller said.

Some immigrants, she added, avoid COVID-19 testing and contact tracing because they are afraid they might be deported.

The result is "a pandemic response that breaks, that doesn't work, and that puts everybody at risk," she said. "So it's really important to make sure that the system works for everybody, so that everybody can stay healthy."

Among problems with education, the report said, are language skills, isolation, cultural norms, and other factors that "dramatically compound" the difficulty families face with online schooling.

Parents described technology and technology literacy challenges:

- "The internet speed is not sufficient and is expensive."
- "Not enough internet or computers for all my children at same time, they share and take turns."
- "The District is assuming that everyone knows how to use technology and we don't."
- "I am not able to help my children with their schoolwork."

In the families Mengistu interviewed, she said parents told her they "have no idea what technology even looks like, for the most part...so they're lost on what to do and how to help their kids." They are wondering, she said, "How do I go back and check they're doing their homework?"

Refugee families also talked about the tough settings in which their children are trying to attend remote school and how hard it is to get help. They don't have quiet places to do their schoolwork, and families aren't always skilled enough in English or familiar enough with the education system to ask for help or understand what help they do have.

The survey also found that most parents, 85%, said their children are not getting enough support with online learning, but 71% said they feel supported by their school and have adequate resources.

The report said the coalition is working now with the San Diego Unified School District to address these concerns.

Lonely and Disoriented

The temporary closures of religious and community organizations also left refugees unmoored, Mengistu said. This was not just because those were social hubs, but because that's where people went to get information and support before the pandemic.

"In our community, people go to faith-based organizations to get community members to talk to, to get help in whatever way they need. Not being able to go to church or a mosque to seek out help was tough for the community," Mengistu said.

Put simply, she said: "Humans need humans."

While 80% of those surveyed said they had at least one source of support to help them cope with the pandemic—often a spouse, friend, or refugee organization—71% said they were worried about their ability to connect to friends and their community.

Like with the Karen refugees, the uncertainty has been hard on the families Mengistu spoke with.

"A lot of families come here so that their kids can have a better future," she said. "So seeing what they see and the difficulties that they themselves are now facing, I think they think, 'What else awaits our children?' You know what I mean? The unknown is definitely scary for them."

With her organization's offices in the College–Rolando area temporarily closed, the nonprofit now offers weekly remote tutoring for kids. The group also has given emergency grants to help people pay their rent.

"One of the great things about the community is that they're very resilient," Mengistu said. "They are people that came from hardship to make a better life for themselves, so it's do or die for them here. They're gonna make a way, one way or another. If it's together or by themselves, they're gonna do it."

rent relief

Cody Dulaney
Low-Income Tenants in San Diego County Can Get 100% of Past-Due Rent Erased

> *This story was originally produced and published by inewsource, a nonprofit, nonpartisan newsroom in San Diego committed to exposing wrongdoing and holding powerful people and institutions accountable. As part of their commitment to keeping the San Diego community informed, inewsource has allowed this story to be reprinted and shared here with you. To learn more about their work and how you can support their journalism, visit inewsource.org.*

July 16, 2021

By the end of this week, eligible tenants in the San Diego region will start seeing 100% of past-due rents erased from the beginning of the pandemic through the end of September.

A new state law that extends eviction protections also allows local agencies to cover all back rent due for low-income tenants impacted by COVID-19.

This comes after news organizations across the state, including inewsource, reported low participation rates for rental and utility assistance programs, which left millions of dollars unspent.

Previously, eligible applicants could only receive 80% of past-due rent, and landlords had to agree to waive the rest. Records show that the landlords of more than 1,000 households throughout San Diego County didn't participate.

State officials hope that erasing all rental debt will increase the number of applications and the amount of money going out the door. It's exactly what tenants and landlords have been calling for.

Even so, some wonder if September 30—when eviction protections expire—will buy enough time for those who have been struggling for the past 16 months.

The ongoing relief efforts have been moving at a snail's pace, thanks largely to bureaucratic red tape and the time it takes to process applications. Now, the region stands to receive at least $112.8 million in additional federal coronavirus aid. That doesn't include the $211 million in state and federal funding received earlier this year, and only 25% of that money has been spent, according to the most recent data available.

"That's a huge amount of money to move in a very short amount of time," said Lucinda Lilley, president of the Southern California Rental Housing Association.

More than 700,000 California households are behind on rent, with each household racking up about $4,400 in debt on average, according to the research firm PolicyLink.

A local jobs report published last month revealed 102,100 people in the San Diego region were still unemployed in mid-April, more than double the pre-pandemic figures. And although an eviction moratorium has kept people in their homes, rental debt has continued to pile up in a county where census data shows nearly half of all housing units are occupied by renters.

So far, roughly 13,000 households throughout San Diego County have already received rental assistance, totaling more than $54.3 million in relief, according to the most recent data available.

The city and county of San Diego started sending payments last week to those that already qualified to erase all rental debt through September 30. Chula Vista will start this week.

Bridging the Gap

Earlier this year, California legislators passed a law, SB 91, that aimed to incentivize landlords to participate with rent relief efforts and keep people in their homes during the pandemic.

The state offered to pay 80% of any rent owed from April 2020 through the end of March 2021, if landlords agreed to waive the rest. If they refuse, eligible tenants would receive a payment for 25% of their rental debt over the same period and still be protected from eviction.

The county and cities of San Diego and Chula Vista received a total of $211 million from the state and federal government because the aid was based on population. All three were accepting applications by mid-March.

But it took roughly two months to process applications and send payments. And records show that some landlords still weren't participating with programs in the county and San Diego:

- Nearly 1 out of every 3 landlords who didn't accept money from the county have a tenant living in El Cajon ZIP codes.
- In San Diego, 1 out of every 4 tenants with resistant landlords were living in ZIP codes in downtown, Mid-City, or City Heights.
- About 1 in 10 San Diego households that didn't receive full payment had landlords who weren't willing to waive 20% of the rental debt.
- More than half of those households in San Diego had a landlord who never responded to officials about the program.

The new law, AB 832, aims to fix this. Now, local agencies can send money to erase all rental debt for eligible households from April 2020 through September 30, making landlords whole and buying much needed time for low-income tenants.

"It feels like the governor is recognizing our role as housing providers and the sacrifices we've had to make," said Lilley, with the Rental Housing Association.

The vast majority of rental property owners who declined to participate didn't do it for nefarious reasons, she added. They either didn't understand the program or didn't want to accept anything other than the full amount owed. Everyone is under a lot of stress, she said.

"Think about what they're trying to navigate right now," Lilley said of property owners who haven't been able to collect rent. "They've got mortgages to pay. They've got insurance to pay. They've got utilities to pay to continue to provide housing. Could their communication [with tenants] come across as abrupt? I would imagine."

Lilley said she suspects this new law, coupled with robust outreach, will make all the difference.

In fact, officials with the city and county of San Diego said they have stepped up outreach efforts.

The San Diego Housing Commission, which oversees the city's program, provided information at multiple community events last month and partnered with a nonprofit, Mid-City CAN, to raise awareness through door knocking and phone calls, said spokesperson Scott Marshall.

In addition to attending outreach events in the community, county officials have also contracted with six community organizations to help tenants and landlords with the application process, said spokesperson Michael Workman.

"I Probably Wouldn't Be Alive"

While the new law does buy more time for low-income tenants, the application process takes so long it might not be enough, said Grace Martinez, director of San Diego's Alliance of Californians for Community Empowerment.

Tenants are still going several weeks without any word on the status of their applications, she said. People are exhausted with the process and landlords are wondering when they will get their money, asking for anything tenants can afford.

"Some tenants don't have anything and they're having to choose between food and rent," Martinez said, adding that people still haven't had an opportunity to catch up.

Genea Wall says that's the situation she's in. The City Heights tenant is a licensed insurance agent who said she has been receiving unemployment benefits since last June. The rent on her two-bedroom, two-bath apartment costs $2,000 a month, but she has to keep the lights on, food in the refrigerator, and gas in her car to get to and from medical appointments.

Wall has Type 2 diabetes, and the stress of this year has affected her health, causing blisters to form on her feet. But things are starting to turn around, she said.

The San Diego Housing Commission covered 80% of her past-due rent in May, totaling $8,000, and she stands to have the rest taken care of through September 30.

Receiving the rent relief, as well as following the doctor's orders and having a positive mindset, has greatly improved her situation, and her wounds are starting to heal, she said.

"If I had to do this on the street, I probably wouldn't be alive," she said, adding that she would definitely face amputation. "You can't keep wounds clean if you're living on the streets."

Cody Dulaney

Hundreds Missed Out on Rent Relief When Landlords Didn't Take the Money

> *This story was originally produced and published by inewsource, a nonprofit, nonpartisan newsroom in San Diego committed to exposing wrongdoing and holding powerful people and institutions accountable. As part of their commitment to keeping the San Diego community informed, inewsource has allowed this story to be reprinted and shared here with you. To learn more about their work and how you can support their journalism, visit inewsource.org.*

March 30, 2021

The city and county of San Diego set aside more than $47 million in federal coronavirus aid last fall to pay landlords whose low-income tenants were behind on rent.

But some eligible renters didn't get any help because their landlords didn't take the money, and they weren't required to explain why.

Public records obtained by inewsource show 1,268 eligible households were denied assistance from the county's rent relief program because their landlords either refused to participate or missed deadlines. The city's program, overseen by the San Diego Housing Commission, had 19 households with landlords who wouldn't accept payments, an agency spokesperson said.

Now, more than $211 million in state and federal funds have poured into the region to help low-income renters. And under a new state law, this time the programs come with built-in incentives designed to persuade landlords to take the money.

Participating landlords would have to accept 80% of any rent owed since April through the end of this month and would have to waive the rest that is owed. If they refuse, eligible tenants would receive a payment for 25% of their rental debt over the same period. As long as tenants use that money to pay their landlord, they would still be protected from eviction until June 30—when a state moratorium is scheduled to expire.

Under the new law, landlords would be required to accept an eligible tenant's payment of 25%, said Debra Carlton, an executive with the California Apartment Association, the state's largest landlord group.

"I don't know what landlord would ever disagree with taking the 80%," Carlton said, adding it's the most any landlord could expect to collect at this point in the pandemic.

Grace Martinez, director of San Diego's Alliance of Californians for Community Empowerment, said if a landlord refuses to participate this time around, they most likely just want the tenant gone. And some aren't waiting for the moratorium to end before trying to evict their tenants, she said.

That appears to be the case for Patty Mendoza, an Imperial Beach renter and an outspoken member of the alliance. She was laid off from her non-emergency medical transport job in April, and the mother of two quickly fell behind in her rent.

Last fall, she qualified for the county's rent relief program, and the most recent payment to her landlord was a $3,000 check sent in December.

Since then, her apartment building changed ownership, and she has missed three more rent payments. Her new landlord sent her a "60-day notice of termination of tenancy," giving her until April 10 to move out, so renovations could be done. With the state moratorium in effect, that's unlikely to happen.

Multiple messages from inewsource to her landlord, Gustavo Verdin, were not returned.

Mendoza has applied for the county's latest program, but she fears her landlord won't participate.

The single mom's monthly rent for a two-bedroom, one-bath apartment is $1,500. A few Marilyn Monroe prints decorate her living room walls, and one giant "Stop All Evictions" banner faces the entryway.

She shares the apartment with her 17-year-old daughter and 10-year-old son, who are attending school online.

Before COVID-19 hit San Diego County a year ago, Mendoza said she was earning $2,000 a month from her job. Now she collects less than $200 a month in unemployment benefits, while continuing to receive $455 a month in child support. She's had to rely on local food pantries to feed her family every week, while rent and utility bills pile up.

Although she applies for jobs, she said she hasn't been able to find work. Even if she did, Mendoza said she worries her asthma would put her at risk for severe illness if she were infected with the virus.

Mendoza said she's tired of seeing her kids cry, wondering where they'll live come April 10.

Her son, she said, often asks: "Mommy, where are we going to go? Mommy, where are we going to put all our stuff? Mommy, what's going to happen to my bed?

"Like, what do you tell your kid?"

Some Landlords Wouldn't Participate

The average California household with unemployed workers has accumulated nearly $4,500 in rental debt through 2020, according to research released in January from the state's nonpartisan Legislative Analyst's Office. The situation could have been worse if local governments hadn't used federal coronavirus aid last year to fund rental assistance programs.

The local programs weren't perfect—San Diego's was rife with delays, and the county sent money to ineligible cities. Even with those problems, the money helped thousands of renters with their rent.

The county spent $27 million assisting more than 10,100 households with rent, records show. The city helped more than 3,700 households with $13.7 million. Both the tenant and the landlord had to cooperate and provide documentation to receive the assistance.

But in some cases, landlords pushed back against both programs. Seventeen landlords declined to work with the city. When that happened, the San Diego Housing Commission used $78,000 in private donations to send payments directly to the renters, agency spokesperson Scott Marshall said.

In the county, nearly 1,240 landlords didn't participate in the program. More than 75% missed the deadline to register for the program or provide the required documents to receive the money, data shows. But 285 landlords outright declined. County officials instead sent those payments to other eligible households, spokesperson Michael Workman said.

The city and county won't release the names of the landlords, citing privacy reasons.

Lucinda Lilley, president of the Southern California Rental Housing Association, suspects those who didn't participate just didn't have the time to jump through the necessary hoops.

She and others in the industry prefer the term "housing provider" rather than "landlord." For many of them, she said, renting out homes isn't a full-time endeavor.

"It's something that they do in addition to their job...to make ends meet," said Lilley, who is also vice president of a property management company. She said she relied on her accounting department to navigate the system for tenants.

Rental property owners have been categorized as "eviction hungry business owners," Lilley said, but that's really not the case.

"We need to, as housing providers, be willing to continue to house individuals and families, and support our communities," she said. "Not to say that we believe that that should be done for free, by any stretch of the imagination."

Some people haven't received a rent payment from tenants since the pandemic began, she said, and they're still expected to maintain the property and pay the mortgage.

Rent Relief Is "Like a Gift"

The economic calamity that COVID-19 has caused is not easing for many people.

A SANDAG report published this month found that about one in four people working jobs in San Diego County that don't require a college education are still unemployed. And though the eviction moratorium has kept people in their homes, rental debt piled up in a county where census data shows nearly half of all housing units are occupied by renters.

That's why California legislators passed the law in January to incentivize landlords. Using the latest round of federal assistance, the state aims to accomplish two things: erase all rental debt for eligible low-income tenants through the end of this month and give landlords most of what they are owed.

The county and cities of San Diego and Chula Vista received the assistance because the aid was based on population. Tenants and landlords could begin submitting applications for the funds this month.

The new programs go beyond covering rent. They also help tenants with utility bills and other household expenses. There's also a possibility that a portion of future rent will be covered if money is still available.

This time, tenants also won't be asked about their citizenship, which means undocumented or mixed-status families can apply for rent relief.

That's a big deal, said Roberto Alcantar, chief strategy officer with the Chicano Federation, one of more than a dozen nonprofits the San Diego

Housing Commission contracted with to help people apply for the city's program.

These changes, coupled with increased funding and resources for outreach, have made a difference, Alcantar said. More people are eligible to apply this time, and more people know how to access it, he said.

Tenants were the ones applying for rent relief last fall, but now landlords are also reaching out to collect what they are owed, said Brenda Aguirre, a family resources navigator with the Chicano Federation.

Lilley with the Southern California Rental Housing Association said that for property owners the promise of collecting 80% of a tenant's back rent is "like a gift, because otherwise there's virtually no chance that they'd ever recover that."

Still, she acknowledges that not all landlords will want to participate.

"We all know those people who have a very strong sense of right and wrong, and to feel like they have been taken advantage of is not an option," she said of accepting anything less than the full amount.

Martinez, who advocates for renters, said tenants across the region are being intimidated into leaving their homes because of questionable 60-day eviction notices. She said that's what's happening to Mendoza, the single mom in Imperial Beach.

Inewsource reached the property manager Mendoza has been dealing with over her eviction notice. He insisted she isn't being evicted, and the owner is working with lawyers on the matter. He declined to comment further and would not give his name.

Mendoza knows she doesn't have to immediately leave her apartment because even tenants with the most resistant landlords are protected until eviction moratoriums expire.

Cody Dulaney
Against Supervisors' Wishes, County Sent Rent Relief Money to Ineligible Cities

> *This story was originally produced and published by inewsource, a nonprofit, nonpartisan newsroom in San Diego committed to exposing wrongdoing and holding powerful people and institutions accountable. As part of their commitment to keeping the San Diego community informed, inewsource has allowed this story to be reprinted and shared here with you. To learn more about their work and how you can support their journalism, visit inewsource.org.*

February 1, 2021

A $27 million rental assistance program the county Board of Supervisors launched in August was supposed to help 10,000 low-income families impacted by COVID-19 who had nowhere else to turn.

Greg Cox and Nathan Fletcher, the two supervisors leading the region's fight against the coronavirus at the time, stressed that the $27 million shouldn't benefit tenants in cities with money in their own rent relief programs.

But that's exactly what happened.

An inewsource analysis of ZIP code data shows roughly three-quarters of the county's money spent through December went to help residents in San Diego, El Cajon, Chula Vista, and La Mesa—cities that had rent relief programs and money still to spend.

Nearly half of the households that received help from the county live in San Diego.

For reasons the county would not explain, staff went against the supervisors' stated wishes and created a standard that ultimately allowed residents in those cities to qualify for the program.

But the standard was not applied across the board.

Tenants in Carlsbad, Escondido, National City, and San Marcos, which also had rent relief programs, were not eligible. Officials in National City and Escondido are crying foul.

"If we were excluded, other cities with their own openly available programs should have been excluded as well out of fairness," said Carlos Aguirre, director of the National City Housing Authority.

National City has been among the hardest hit by unemployment during the pandemic, and the city's mayor, Alejandra Sotelo-Solis, said all of the county's COVID-19 resources should be based on need.

"I think there needs to be that deeper dive in how those resources are being distributed," Sotelo-Solis said.

Mike Strong, Escondido's Community Development director, said he wants answers from the county about why this happened.

"I think the end goal is to make sure that any eligible recipient, regardless of jurisdiction, is afforded access to the same opportunities," Strong said.

Last week, the Board of Supervisors approved a new $49 million aid package that goes beyond covering rent. It also helps people with utility and other household expenses. The money comes from federal coronavirus funds.

Expected to roll out this month, the new program will exclude residents in San Diego and Chula Vista because those cities also have received federal aid for these purposes.

But none of this changes the program the supervisors approved in August. Fletcher said at last week's board meeting the original program still has $13 million to be spent.

Inewsource attempted several times to interview Fletcher, now the board chairman, about how the first program unfolded and how he plans to ensure this new one rolls out as intended. His spokesperson did not respond to those interview requests.

A county spokesperson also did not respond to questions about why staffers didn't follow the board's directive with the first program.

"Badly Needed" Program

COVID-19 has led to the highest unemployment level since the Great Depression, causing nearly 90,000 California households to fall behind in rent, according to research released last month from the state's nonpartisan Legislative Analyst's Office.

The average California household with unemployed workers has accumulated nearly $4,500 in rental debt, the study said, and it could have been worse if cities and counties hadn't created rental assistance programs. Much of the money came from federal coronavirus aid and was based on population.

That meant unincorporated areas and small cities relied on San Diego County for help.

The county's $27 million rent relief program started with an August 19 letter from Cox and Fletcher requesting a change to the county's budget.

It stated plainly: "Residents who live within jurisdictions with their own COVID-19 rental relief program would not be eligible for the County program unless those jurisdictions' funds have already been depleted."

At a board meeting to discuss the proposal, then-Supervisor Dianne Jacob, who represented East County for 28 years before leaving office last month, said the program was "badly needed." She asked that priority be given to the 2,000 renters in unincorporated areas who "are on the list, ready to go."

"I don't know how staff is going to work out priorities, but I want to make sure that these folks are taken care of," Jacob said.

The measure passed the five-member board unanimously.

But a month later, county staff overseeing the program changed which areas would be eligible.

Residents were excluded from the county's program only if their city had a rent relief program that was accepting or planning to accept applications at the same time as the county, Michael Workman, a county spokesperson told inewsource in an email. Because San Diego was not accepting applications, their residents qualified for the county program, Workman said.

He did not address why money went to the cities of Chula Vista, El Cajon, or La Mesa, and when inewsource told him those cities still had money available for their residents, he offered no explanation. He also didn't respond to requests to interview the person in charge of the county's program.

Through December, the county had spent $10.9 million helping more than 4,000 households. About 330 of those are in unincorporated areas, representing about 980 people based on SANDAG's average household estimates. That's far fewer than what Jacob had hoped for.

Tenants in Some Cities Had Two Safety Nets

The county's implementation plan shows that staffers were supposed to consider two things when gauging a city's eligibility for the rent relief program: the application period and whether money was still available to help tenants.

Using that criteria, San Diego renters shouldn't have been eligible for the county's program. San Diego still had more than $9 million in rental assistance when the county started accepting applications in September, according to San Diego Housing Commission records.

The Housing Commission has also been sitting on another $5 million that was approved in October to help renters and has not said when it will spend the money. Mayor Todd Gloria also announced last month a new $42 million rental assistance program.

Meanwhile, the county has spent $4.9 million on rent relief for 1,860 San Diego households.

County spokesperson Workman contended in emails that San Diego residents were eligible for the county's program all along. But Housing Commission spokesperson Scott Marshall disputes that. He said city residents weren't eligible for the county's program until December 1.

By that time, the city's program had run out of money, which made city residents eligible, Marshall said. But that's not the complete picture.

Marshall revealed—after inewsource obtained emails between the commission and tenants' landlords—that the agency continued in December to provide more than $100,000 in rent relief from unused administrative costs.

So far, the city's program, which was rife with delays, has helped more than 3,700 San Diego households with about $13.7 million, Marshall said.

Concern About Inequity in County Program

Officials in Escondido and National City said they're left wondering why their renters were excluded from the county's multimillion-dollar program.

National City housing official Aguirre said his city wanted to help struggling renters during the pandemic, so officials put together a $558,000 program from various funding sources before the county's program began.

The City Council approved it in mid-August. Because that money had been set aside, National City residents were ineligible for the county's rent relief, he said.

The same issue initially excluded Escondido renters from applying for the county program.

Escondido had created a $268,000 rental assistance program from a variety of sources, but tenants weren't eligible to apply for the aid until they received an eviction notice, said Karen Youel, the city's Housing and Neighborhood Services manager. With the state's moratorium on evictions in place, the city's program wasn't running.

Because Escondido had money available—even though it couldn't be spent—county officials excluded those residents, said Strong, the city's community development director.

Escondido put its program on hold in mid-November so residents could qualify for county money.

An inewsource analysis found that at most 109 Escondido households received about $295,000 in rental assistance from the county through the end of December.

Escondido Mayor Paul McNamara told inewsource he is "concerned about what appears to be an inequity" in how the county program worked, and he will ask city staff to investigate.

Just before leaving the Board of Supervisors in January, Cox suggested that the county's program didn't roll out as it was intended.

"We did say that residents who live in cities with their own COVID-19 rental relief program would not be eligible for the County program, unless their cities' funds had already been depleted," Cox said in an email to inewsource. "We hope this program can help as many people as possible during this difficult time."

Inewsource investigative data reporter Jill Castellano and web producer/reporter Bella Ross contributed to this story

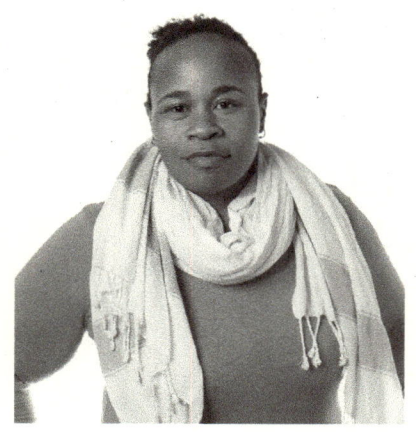

Lindsay Hood, an award-winning journalist who has been shaping the narrative in San Diego since 2004, boasts a diverse background in both print and television journalism. With a bachelor's degree in American Studies from San Diego State University, a Masters of Business Administration from the University of Redlands, and a Masters of Science in Human-Computer Interaction from Iowa State University, Hood's academic prowess is matched only by her passion for storytelling. Her journey into journalism was solidified during her visit to the Newseum in Washington D.C., where she realized the profound impact of documenting history through journalism. Throughout her career, Hood has garnered numerous accolades and awards for her storytelling skills.

A journalist deeply connected to her native San Diego, Hood's latest endeavor, "Stories of San Diego," is a testament to her commitment to giving back to her community. By assembling a team of world-class journalists, she ensures that stories are told authentically and comprehensively, without compromise. Through her leadership, Hood continues to inspire others to recognize the power of storytelling in shaping a more inclusive society.